herbal remedies

how to make, use and grow them

Sorrell Robbins

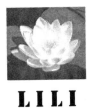

L I L I

Published in December 2007 by

Low-Impact Living Initiative
Redfield Community,
Winslow, Bucks, MK18 3LZ, UK
+44 (0)1296 714184

lili@lowimpact.org
www.lowimpact.org

ISBN 978-0-9549171-4-2

Illustrations: Perdita Robbins

Printed in Great Britain by
Lightning Source, Milton Keynes

important note
The information contained in this book is intended as a general guide to using plants and is not comprehensive or specific to individuals or their particular circumstances. Many plant substances, whether sold as foods or medicines, and used internally or externally, can cause an allergic reaction in some people. Some plants are toxic if taken in large quantities or over a long period of time. Others may have an unpleasant effect in specific circumstances. Neither the author nor the publishers can be held responsible for claims arising from the inappropriate use of any remedy or healing regime. Do not attempt self-diagnosis or self-treatment for serious or long-term conditions before consulting a medical professional or qualified practitioner. Do not undertake any self-treatment while taking other prescribed drugs or receiving therapy without first seeking professional guidance. Always seek medical advice if any symptoms persist.

contents

about the author

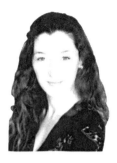

Sorrell has been a health practitioner since 1996 and has several professional qualifications including a BSc (Hons) in Herbal Medicine, diplomas in Clinical Aromatherapy and Therapeutic Massage, Advanced Hypnotherapy and Hypnohealing, and Advanced Reiki. She has undertaken many post-graduate, advanced courses in both herbal medicine and massage and also studies shamanic healing.

She devised and teaches the Herbal Medicine course for the Low-Impact Living Initiative (LILI). The main aim of the course is to give beginners the basic skills and knowledge to enable them to use herbal medicine safely and effectively in everyday life with herbs from familiar and readily-available sources. She also teaches for Thames Valley University and the Institute of Traditional Herbal Medicine and Aromatherapy, and devised and wrote an online course, called Introductory Course in Aromatherapy, for Learndirect.

Sorrell is passionate about using complementary medicine techniques to assist people in recovering from ill health and helping them learn how to use these techniques to stay healthy. She runs busy practices in London and Hertfordshire using all of her chosen disciplines. When she isn't busy teaching or consulting you will find her in her herb garden in south-east London where she grows medicinal herbs, makes traditional medicines and distils her own essential oils.

Sorrell can be contacted at sorrellrobbins@gmail.com.

herbal remedies: how to make, use and grow them **L I L I**

introduction

This book aims to get you excited and inspired about using herbs, to give you the knowledge to use them effectively and to help build your confidence to experiment with new ways of using them. You may wish to grow your own herbs, use them as medicines for yourself and your family's health, or just to bring some new knowledge of herbs into your kitchen where your salads will suddenly be coloured with Borage flowers, your biscuits flavoured with Lavender and your cocktails infused with aphrodisiac Damaina. Or perhaps you want to know how to treat coughs and colds using the herb and spice rack and the lemons in the fruit dish. You may want to know how herbs can help you reduce the symptoms of more chronic conditions such as arthritis or irritable bowel syndrome, ME or insomnia. Wherever your interest stems from, getting to know the herbs in this book will show you new ways to enjoy herbs and teach you how to use them to become healthier and to maintain your health. Herbs are here to make our lives better, to help us feel good in our bodies and happy to be alive. They have the potential to make us physically and emotionally well and to help us really enjoy life.

I hope the book will also change the way you see the world around you. Wherever you walk, not just those of you who live in the country but city dwellers too, you are surrounded by herbal medicines. On every patch of waste ground, in every park, in the cracks in the pavement, in the patch of lawn in your garden those weeds, which we normally ignore or try to eradicate, will suddenly be seen as respected medicines with powerful chemical properties to utilise for the herbal medicine cabinet. The book will also enable you to go to your kitchen cupboard, to your spice rack, to shop at your grocery store or supermarket and have the knowledge to make remedies for many common ailments, whether they are physical, mental or emotional.

It will provide you with all the basics you need to start growing your own herbs regardless of the size of your garden. Herbs are ideal for a novice gardener as they are incredibly tolerant, generally preferring not to be fussed over too much. It will guide you in the methods to use for collecting, drying and storing your own herbs, whether they are home grown, from the weed patch in the garden or collected from the wild.

how to use this book

The book is divided into several sections and you can read it cover to cover or dip in and out as you like. There are recipes and ideas to enthuse you throughout the book and I would like to encourage you to try them and see for yourself how herbs really work.

Firstly we guide you through the different types of herbal preparations; from teas to tinctures, essential oils to herbal infused oils. We look at their differences and similarities and explain how to choose one preparation over another in response to your needs.

We then take a moment to introduce you to each system of the body individually so you can understand how and why things go wrong with them. This will enable you to develop an ability to choose how to treat the root of any health problem in a particular area of the body. We also show you how all these systems are linked to each other so you can learn to judge how other body systems may be affected by the original condition and know how to treat them. We also explain the terminology generally used to describe the body systems within herbal medicine text books so you can also use other books more easily. The properties of herbs related to these systems are described, along with the precautions you should take to be safe and effective in your choices. Each body system has a separate section detailing herbs, and combinations of herbs, to use to get you started on treating different conditions and ailments affecting that body system.

After the body system section are forty-four herb monographs describing common herbs you can grow, collect from the wild or buy in local shops. There are over two thousand herbs used in European herbal medicine, so this list is far from complete! It is however, more than enough for you to be able to begin your journey and be really effective in your treatments. By using an exclusive range of herbs, and those readily available to you, you can get to know this selection of herbs really well and understand how best to use them to treat a whole number of common complaints and conditions. There is just one herb included which is a little more difficult to find in Europe as it is harvested from the deserts of Africa. It is Myrrh and, once as precious as gold, its properties are so unique and powerfully therapeutic it had to be included. I find Myrrh constantly useful in the treatment of so many ailments and I think it is worth the extra effort needed to source it from more specialist shops.

Once you have got to know the tools of the trade more intimately we get really practical and show you how to make your own herbal medicine preparations, from teas to creams and ointments, from wines to herbal honeys. This practical medicine-making section contains lots and lots of recipes for you to try out and start to get hands-on with. This is where the fun really starts and your confidence in using herbs can begin to grow.

We then give you an introduction to the fascinating world of growing herbs, offering advice on how to get going and some designs and planting schemes which can be adapted to any size of garden.

The very last section is all about gathering, preparing for storage and how to store herbs so you maximise their therapeutic properties.

We hope you enjoy the journey this book takes you on and that it inspires you to get more intimate with herbs, have fun and benefit from using them every day.

My aim in writing this book is to offer you a way to begin, and become confident in, using herbs even if you have no previous experience. It gently walks you through all the stages you need to begin to understand your own body better and then shows you how to choose the right herbs for your individual purpose. There are guidelines for dosage, suggestions on how to blend herbs together and a multitude of recipes and ideas for you to try. You will never be short of inspiration with this book in your hands!

what is herbal medicine?

Herbal medicine is the use of medicinal plants to treat disease, and to restore and maintain health. It is the oldest known form of medicine and is still relied upon by eighty per cent of the world's population, according to World Health Organisation figures. With the combination of thousands of years of documented use and modern research techniques we are now able to understand how and why plant medicines are effective and to use them to an exceptional standard of knowledge and skill.

why herbal medicine is effective

By using the appropriate plant medicines we are able to treat the cause of ill heath and at the same time alleviate the symptoms. Herbs can help to restore the correct functioning, strength and balance of all the body's systems where they have become weakened.

Herbs can be thought of as food feeding specific elements of our physical body: they work at a chemical and cellular level and can activate certain processes innate within us, which may just need a little stimulus to bring them up to their full potential. These processes can be detoxifying, for example by stimulating the elimination of toxic chemicals causing irritation such as uric acid crystals locked in joints which produce the painful condition known as gout. They can build, encouraging the repair of tissues; like Comfrey which speeds up cell regeneration and enables faster repair of damaged tissues. Through their action the body can fight disease and regain health. Or they can stimulate the immune system to attack pathogens when we have been invaded by flu or cold bugs.

Plant medicines are powerful and some basic knowledge is required to choose the appropriate herb or blend of herbs for the right purpose. When used correctly, at a suitable dose, plant medicines are extremely effective, safe and free from side effects.

the holistic approach

By choosing to use a natural form of medicine it is easy to assume that you will also be drawn to the holistic approach. This term describes an approach which looks not only at the symptomatology of a disease but also at the wider perspective in an attempt to find the cause of the problem. It includes looking at the individual's lifestyle, their diet, their physical activities, their social activities, and their mental, spiritual and emotional health. All these elements contribute to a person's wellbeing and state of health. If any one of these elements is ignored when trying to treat a health concern the cause of the problem may be overlooked and the problem may not resolve even with the best choice of medicines.

Herbs can treat symptoms and heal the cause in many situations. However, herbal medicine can not always touch the elements of people's lives which need to change in order for them to heal. In this situation herbal medicine can be used to support the healing process but the changes may have to come in another form.

when to use herbal medicines

Herbs can be used to prevent ill health and maintain wellbeing on a daily basis, safely and for free. If you know you have general weakness in one area of the body, or would simply like to support and tone that part, you can choose a herb to feed that area, for example nettle for simple iron-deficiency anaemia, raspberry leaf to maintain the health of the reproductive organs and prepare for a speedy delivery at childbirth.

Herbs can be used for culinary purposes, nettles in place of spinach for example: or aromatic herbs in Italian cooking and Dandelion leaves in salads. Many of the herbs used in this country are thought of as vegetables elsewhere in world, such as Cleavers and Burdock root, which are eaten as vegetables in China.

Herbs can also be used to treat health problems once they have occurred. It is always worth seeking professional help when suffering any health problem whether physical or otherwise.

However, with simple, easily-defined illnesses we can do a lot for ourselves and, up to a couple of hundred years ago it would have been standard practice to do so. Somehow the knowledge was wiped out of general circulation to become the property of a select few, and for no apparently good reason as this form of medicine is generally very safe, gentle and really works!

self-prescribing: choosing the right herbs for you

There are more than two thousand herbs in use in European traditional herbal medicine so how do you know whether a herb is really the right one when there are so many to choose from?

Herbs can take time to be effective and one of the basic things you have to consider is how long you continue to use a herb before trying another or consulting a professional practitioner. In traditional herbal medicine we work on the premise that for each year you have had a condition it will take one month for it to begin to be healed using herbs. That also means the longer you leave it the harder it is to get well. It is obvious that most acute conditions like a common cold should heal more quickly than more chronic conditions such as arthritis. However, a chronic condition such as ME may set in following a respiratory infection or arthritis may be acute, mild and short-lived if it is treated at the onset. So there are variables in every field and each case should be looked at individually. With most conditions I use the basic rule that I want to see changes within one month of using a herb or herbal formula. Most of the time improvements are seen much faster. The changes may be small, such as improved sleeping patterns or better digestion, or may appear more significant such as increased mobility or perhaps relief from symptoms of anxiety or depression. Some body systems, such as the endocrine system in women, take longer to show up healing changes. This is because the endocrine system works more slowly on monthly cycles and I would expect to wait from three to six months to notice any real changes in the hormonal system of female clients.

when to contact a medical herbalist

If you are on any medication, if you are pregnant or attempting to get pregnant, if you have any chronic disease symptoms, if you need help defining your illness or choosing the right herbs for your health condition consult a professional medical herbalist. Self-diagnosis is never easy; if a medical herbalist is not available then consult a GP or other professional healthcare advisor so you can have a better idea of what you are dealing with and how to approach it effectively.

When you are looking for a good medical herbalist there are several registers you can try to ensure they are qualified to the appropriate standard. The National Institute of Medical Herbalists has a great website which leads you to your local herbalist: www.NIMH.org.uk.

a cautionary note

When you are using herbs for any purpose it is always worth bearing in mind that they are powerful biochemical medicines. As long as you use the appropriate dosage and avoid using herbs which are contraindicated for a particular condition they are extremely safe. Please also be aware that essential oils are very concentrated and should not be ingested at all unless directed by a medical herbalist.

Please check any herb's contraindication before using it unless you are familiar with its use already.

This precaution is especially pertinent during pregnancy and breastfeeding as herbs which affect the mother will be passed on to the child via the placenta or breast milk. Sometimes this is beneficial, for example, using Fennel seed for colic in babies is extremely effective if the mother adds Fennel tea to her diet and the power of the herb is passed on to the baby via the breast milk. However, sometimes avoidance of certain herbs is advisable. For example, some herbs like Sage, Wormwood and Thyme have a high percentage of a chemical called ketones in their make-up, which can act as a nerve tonic in low dose but as a nerve toxin in excess. Care should be taken with such herbs; they can be ingested in food but they should not be used at a higher, medicinal dosage.

Very rarely a person may have allergic reactions to or intolerances of some individual herbs in the same way as others have allergic hayfever, eczema or react to some foodstuffs. If this occurs consult a medical professional and stop using the herb concerned.

If you are ever in doubt please check this book, or another respected publication, for clarification on the individual guidelines for each herb. And remember, as long as you follow those guidelines you will be safe and effective in using herbs.

a short history of herbal medicine

We probably all have our own experiences with medicinal herbs and knowledge passed on to us by our parents, grandparents, friends or local herbalist. Most of us still drink lemon and honey when we have a cold or enjoy a spicy punch on bonfire night to keep us warm. We may also remember being told by friends or family that Dock leaves relieve nettle stings or that rosehips can be used for their vitamin C content to ward off illness.

Herbal medicine is the oldest form of therapy practised by mankind; so where did it all begin? Where did this knowledge come from? Let's go way back: to Neanderthal man. A grave was recently discovered in Iraq; it was the grave of a Neanderthal man some 60,000 years old. Accompanying his body, in the soil around his bones, were large quantities of pollen grains. These pollens were analysed and found to come from eight plant species which still thrive in the local area and, remarkably, seven of them are still used as medicinal herbs by the local people and herbalists throughout the world. We can only really guess why these particular plants were there but it is generally believed they were chosen for their medicinal benefit: as healing plants to lay with the body perhaps to fortify him on his journey to another world.

There are different theories as to how we first developed our knowledge of herbal medicine. The dowsing instinct is one; an innate ability to seek out plants which may supply nutrients and instinctively avoid those which contain poisons. It is certainly interesting to note that people in different countries with no communication are found to use the same herbs for the same purpose.

Another popular idea is the 'Doctrine of Signatures'; the belief that plants have been created to show what they are good for. For example, yellow plants are often good liver stimulants and can treat jaundice, while Lungwort, with the white patches on its leaves, can be seen to be good for congestion on the lungs.

Before there were written records traditions and knowledge were passed down orally from generation to generation. As civilisations developed systems of written communication were established and methods of treating ill health were written down in Materia Medicas. These provided a record of all the plants, minerals and animal parts used in medicine at the time.

The earliest written Materia Medica is from China. The *Pen Ts'ao* is thought to have been written around 2800 BC by Shen Nung. China was also the first country to develop a system of medicine, between 4000 BC and 2000 BC. It stemmed from the Taoist, Buddhist and Confucianist belief structures, based on the Yin-Yang and Five Elements theories, Qi (pronounced 'chee') energy and applied to establish balance in the individual.

Though Egyptian medicine dates from about 2900 BC its best known, and most important pharmaceutical record, is the *Papyrus Ebers* (1500 BC): a collection of eight hundred prescriptions, mentioning seven hundred drugs, most of which are herbal in origin. It is a compilation of earlier works containing a large number of remedies and prescriptions showing how to treat many disorders using a variety of substances, mostly plant but also animal, mineral and the droppings and urine of various animals.

Greek medicine, as developed by Hippocrates (460–370 BC), thought of as the founder of modern medicine, and Aristotle (384–322 BC), drew on their prevailing philosophical thought; that the world around them was made up of four elements: air, earth, fire and water. They used this theory to devise a system which could classify the human state of health and disease. The fluids, or humours, of the body corresponded to these elements: choleric (yellow bile) linked with fire; sanguine (blood) linked with air; phlegmatic (phlegm) associated with water and melancholic (black bile) linked with earth. Herbs were classified by their effect on the body's four humours and were described as moist, dry, hot or cold.

As with the traditional Chinese system of medicine, the essence of Greek medicine was balance: mental, emotional and physical. Disease was a disturbance of the balance of one or more of the humours and the physician's task was to restore balance with herbs and assist the patient's own natural ability to heal.

Galen was an ambitious Greek physician in the Roman Empire during the second century AD. He developed the humoural system into an even more elaborate system of medicine which was used throughout Europe for the next fifteen centuries. Nobody appears to have questioned the system or thought further on the use of herbs during that time.

Galen's theory and system of medicine was taught to students at medical schools right up until the sixteenth and seventeenth centuries. They learnt how to diagnose an imbalance of the humours and the methods used to re-establish equilibrium. Purging and blood-letting became the most popular ways to treat these imbalances and herbs were used less, almost as a secondary part of treatment.

In the seventh century the Arabs invaded North Africa and the Mediterranean. Greek and Roman medical texts were collected and stored in the 'House of Wisdom' in Baghdad. During the ninth century these works were translated into Arabic and their medical men began to get to grips with the traditional system of Graeco-Roman medicine. The Arabs already had a reputation for producing great doctors but the introduction of this different tradition sparked a huge development in Arabic medicine which was to influence the practice and production of medicine throughout the world.

Avicenna, Mesue and Rhazes are the most remembered characters of this era. They adopted the teachings of Hippocrates and developed teaching hospitals. They paid particular attention to environmental factors involved in disease. They also focused on the study of clinical medicine, the investigation of disease at the sick bed, rather than in the laboratory or lecture hall. Preventative medicine and public health issues were also studied.

The actions of plants were carefully studied, often with cautious experiments on human beings, and the resulting observations of potency, dosage, and possible toxicity were carefully noted in collections of case histories which were then studied at medical schools. By AD 800 pharmacy had become a distinct and separate profession among the Muslims practised by carefully trained specialists. It is thought the first pharmacy shops were opened in Baghdad in the early ninth century. Drugs and spices from Africa and Asia were readily available. Within a short period of time pharmacy shops sprang up in other large cities throughout Europe, especially where proximity to military installations increased the need for medications.

Avicenna (930–1037) took over where Galen left off and through his work confirmed the authority of Galen in the medical world. The typical medieval physician was trained in their style, using astrology, the system of the four humours and urinalysis to form a diagnosis and treatment plan for their patients. This type of physician became known as a 'mouthing' doctor as opposed to the surgeon who was known as the 'wound' doctor.

Soon Arab pharmacy was having an enormous influence on European prescribing habits. The new drugs developed by the Arab pharmacists were taken back to Europe by physicians who travelled with the Crusades.

Another important influence was alchemy, a mix of philosophy and chemistry thought to have originated from Asia during the thirteenth century. Alchemists experimented with the use of minerals in medicine including mercury, which was used extensively to try to treat syphilis.

Paracelsus was an influential sixteenth-century physician and herbalist who renounced the teachings of Galen and Hippocrates, and especially the blind faith modern practitioners had in their methods. He was much keener on the teachings of the old women healers, who had hands-on experience with herbs, than on a text book education. At a time when most physicians were studying herbal medicines on paper alone and within the confines of the humoural approach, Paracelsus went out of his way to study with gypsies and country healers. He also applied alchemy to his herbal preparations, arguing that alchemy offered new possibilities for penetrating the medicinal secrets of plants and using them more effectively. He believed in what is now called the 'active principle' of plants and the 'Doctrine of Signatures'. His actions and approach, ironically, made him a figurehead of the new medical revolution that was bringing chemically-prepared mineral medicines into the apothecary's shop.

herbal medicine in Britain

The systems of Hippocrates and Galen were spread through Britain by the Romans. They also brought plants with them from Europe which they used for treating their army and many of these flourished and spread. When the Roman armies withdrew in AD 407 the plants remained along with some of their physicians.

Before the Romans came to Britain, traditional knowledge of the native healing plants was extensive. In Wales medicine was regarded as one of the three civil arts, together with navigation and commerce. The tradition of priest-healers in Wales can be traced back to 1000 BC.

The Druids studied astrology and theology and were adept at divination, having a deep reverence for the moon which they believed had a powerful influence on both people and plants. They were also skilled in the use of medicinal herbs. Alongside the priest-healers an independent school of physicians, with a rational rather than priestly approach, was established during the late sixteenth century in Myddfai in Wales. Welsh practice was a significant influence on herbal medicine in England, especially in the counties of Herefordshire and Worcestershire.

In AD 597 Christianity arrived in England, bringing with it new traditions of monastic medicine. The Benedictines considered it their duty to care for the sick and to do so as skilfully and intelligently as possible. Every monastery had a physic garden and the monks cared not only for their own sick but also the poor, local people and passing strangers. These doctoring monks can be thought of as amateurs but they worked diligently and over the years developed considerable skill. They trained their own monks and also took on pupils from outside the monastery. Until the first universities were established this was the only form of training available for physicians.

Medically, England may have been ahead of the Continent. The earliest surviving medical text, *the Leech Book of Bald* written in the early tenth century, was a compilation of the best Roman and Greek medical literature available in Europe at that time.

A careful reading of this book shows that Bald had a kindly approach to his patients and there are remedies for the more trivial ailments, such as hangovers, loss of appetite and sleeplessness, suggesting he was writing for a wider audience than the professional physician. The majority of remedies mentioned were herbal.

By the sixteenth century medicine was a popular pastime in England. There was much money to be made especially in London, where overcrowding and lack of sanitation caused ill health and there was long-standing epidemic of syphilis. There was no system of regulation and different schools produced practitioners of varying standards alongside the folk healers, apothecaries and surgeons.

In 1512 Parliament passed a series of Acts designed to regulate the practice of medicine in London and the provinces. The practice of medicine within a seven-mile radius of London was restricted to graduates of Oxford and Cambridge. Six years later this legislation was extended to the whole of England. Later, in 1540, a further act was passed reconfirming the physicians' authority, giving them control over apothecaries and surgeons and giving surgeons authority over barber surgeons.

This new legislation, rather than keeping people safe from the harmful methods of quacks and charlatans, only led to increased problems as the poor were unable to afford the expensive treatments available from the physicians, surgeons and apothecaries. Parliament, aware of this divide and encouraged by the amateur apothecary Henry VIII, acted in 1542 and introduced further legislation to effectively legalise an entirely new class of practitioner: the herbalist. This Act has been known ever since as the Quacks Charter, although herbalists like to call it the Herbalists' Charter!

Interestingly, this charter allows herbalists to treat a far greater number of disorders than the surgeons. It shows that herbalists also had friends in high places, Henry VIII included, and implies that traditional medicine was practised by knowledgeable, honest men and women who provided a much-needed medical service to the poor.

By the seventeenth century professional physicians were few and far between and day-to-day medicine was practised by the 'housewives' of Britain. Herbal recipes were passed down from generation to generation. The vicar's wife would certainly have been responsible for taking care of the sick within her parish.

Killer diseases such as smallpox, the plague, which occurred occasionally until 1665, and tuberculosis, endemic in some parts of the country, were beyond the housewife's ability and professional help would be needed for them. The housewife would be the first port of call though, responsible for the initial diagnosis and the overall care of the sick during convalescence. Wealthier people had the luxury of calling their physician for every complaint although they would be treated with more drastic techniques including mercury, antimony, bleeding and purges.

The housewife chose domestic herbal medicine for simple reasons: the new, imported exotics, like powdered mummy, stag's heart, bone and pearls, were simply too expensive and unpalatable for their patients. And, although England at this time was desperately short of trained doctors, the wealthy members of the College of Physicians did their best not to share the secrets of their medicine. They always printed their works and pharmacopoeias in Latin, which housewives and apothecaries would have been unable to read.

One person who found this attitude ridiculous was Nicholas Culpepper (1616–1654). He studied medicine at Cambridge University but left before completing his degree. He established an apothecary shop in Spitalfields, a poor area of London, and was passionate about working with the poor. Instead of prescribing expensive, imported treatments he prescribed cheap, wholesome, home grown herbs, encouraging people to pick herbs from their own gardens whenever they could.

He was aware that he was advantaged due to his superior education and wanted to raise the overall standard of his profession. As a result, in 1649, he decided to translate the *London Pharmacopoeia* into English so that the 'whole body of physick' was available; he also took the liberty of amending this book where he considered it appropriate. As you can imagine the College of Physicians was not amused and attacked him vigorously.

Culpepper went on to write *The English Physician*, a herbal based on his own method which incorporated astrology. It was an instant success and has continued to be so through the centuries. Culpepper's herbal served to reinforce a strong English tradition for domestic herbal medicine at a time when professional physicians were encouraging contempt for these traditional practices.

During the eighteenth and early nineteenth centuries the nature of British society changed as the effects of the Industrial Revolution took hold. A large proportion of the population was gathered into cities and there were epidemics of typhoid and cholera. Much of the local herbalist's wisdom was lost to the majority of people but during the 1830s the American 'Thomsonian System' was introduced to Britain by Albert Coffin and expanded, though with much conflict, by Dr Wooster Beach and John Skelton. This system combined the use of some of the strongest herbs, like chilli, in teas or as enemas, with the sweating techniques learned from Native American Indians and had proved successful in combating some instances of typhoid and cholera. Unfortunately in Britain these diseases were primarily caused by environmental factors, like bad hygiene and living conditions, at that time and the use of this system proved almost entirely unsuccessful.

Today, even though herbal medicine is arguably the oldest form of medicine used by man, it is, perhaps surprisingly, still the most commonly used across the globe. According to the World Health Organization it is practiced three to four times more frequently than orthodox medicine. Herbs also appear in medicines prescribed by orthodox doctors, albeit in refined forms. There are varying estimates of how many orthodox medicines were developed originally from herbal preparations; the figures I have seen range between twenty and forty per cent of modern medicines used globally. Obvious examples include the development and use of aspirin and codeine for pain relief, hyoscyamine and other alkaloids as antispasmodics and digoxin as a cardiac stimulant.

As history shows there have been a few adversaries trying to ban or restrict the use and practice of herbal medicine in Europe and Britain. Over the years it has been banned and, thankfully, legalized again in Britain and currently the situation is fairly positive. Although some countries in Europe do not allow anyone other than their orthodox, medically-trained doctors to prescribe herbs and essential oil preparations, in Britain a register is being established by the Government in conjunction with leading associations who voluntarily register qualified professionals so that the public will soon have a more reliable system whereby they can find a qualified professional medical herbalist.

No matter what the law dictates, the human race will always have a use for herbs, we will individually always be able to grow our own medicines and take care of ourselves and, at the very least, be able to enhance our wellbeing by making a nice cup of lemon balm tea fresh from the garden.

herbal products

teas

Tea can be made from the fresh or dried herb, from the flowers, leaves or stems of a plant. Dosage is usually about two teaspoons per cup per person. In general it is best to infuse the herb for 10–20 minutes and drink three cups daily. Check the dosage given for individual herbs as some are more potent than others.

decoctions

Decoctions are made from the tougher parts of a plant: roots, bark and berries. The plant matter is brought to the boil and simmered for twenty minutes, then strained. The dosage is usually two teaspoons of plant matter per cup per person; remember to add a little more water than is required as some will evaporate during the process.

tinctures

A tincture is the alcoholic extraction of the active ingredients of the herb and can be made by soaking dried or fresh plant material in a mixture of alcohol and water to various strengths from 25 to 90 per cent alcohol. The highest percentage of alcohol generally available is 45 per cent, in the form of vodka or other spirit. The standard ratio of plant to alcohol is 1:5, which would be, for example, 10g plant matter to 50ml alcohol. This ratio can vary from 2:1 to 1:20 depending on the strength of the herb and the purpose of the tincture being made.

There are different types of tinctures, for example, distilled tinctures, infused tinctures, decocted tinctures, where the water element of the tincture is replaced by an infusion, decoction or the aromatic water in the case of a distilled tincture. These are much stronger than ordinary tinctures and are currently only readily available to medical herbalists, although they are not restricted for sale to the public and you can make them yourself.

fresh juices

Juices are easy to extract from herbs if you have a juicer. These are now readily available at affordable prices and extract very strong, medicinally-active juices from fruit, vegetables and herbs for use as medicines. Juices are a relatively recent discovery in the world of herbal medicine and there is not that much information available about dosage and medicinal value. So I advise careful experimentation; only use herbs which have no contraindications and start with small doses so you can measure your own response to them.

vinegar extracts

Cider and wine vinegars have been used traditionally throughout Europe to produce herbal medicines. They are better for people who do not tolerate alcohol well, like ex-alcoholics, and cider vinegar has its own medicinal benefits.

herbal honeys

Honey is the best preservative on the planet! It lasts forever and is highly anti-microbial, protecting anything contained within it from going mouldy or oxidising. It is also delicious and a very good way of getting medicines into fussy children.

capsules

Capsules and pills are the most common form of herbal product on the shelves of our health food stores and pharmacies. This is fine, although they are probably the most expensive way to take the product. Capsules can be made at home easily and cheaply. The empty capsules are available in vegetarian forms when required. Capsule makers are also available at an affordable price, they take a lot of the strain out of the job and help you to pack more herb in to each capsule. The advantages of capsules are that you don't taste a thing and they are fairly easy to take.

wines & beers

What a delicious way to take medicine: as a glass of wine! Elderberry is the best known classic herbal wine and, although you can make wine out of anything, it is one of the most popular and effective. Recipes for herbal wines and beers are available in the older herbal publications and there are books specifically about the subject, which are well worth purchasing if this subject interests you.

soups, biscuits, salads etc ...

Examples are Lavender shortbread, Nettle and Mallow flower soups - and they are delicious. Nettles can be used as an alternative to spinach in any cooking recipe if you are brave enough to collect them! Dandelion leaves make a very nutritious addition to any salad bowl. Hawthorn used to be called 'bread and cheese' because the leaves and flowers were eaten by travellers to maintain their energy levels en route. Once again the older herbal publications list recipes and others can be found on the Internet.

creams & ointments

Creams and ointments containing medicinal plant extracts are a great way to work on any condition affecting the skin. They can be made in a traditional way, infusing a herb in lard or blending oil and beeswax, or with a more modern approach using refined chemicals, or by simply adding an extract to a commercially-produced base cream. There are many recipes available for making your own ointments and creams and they are well worth experimenting with if you have the time and don't mind lots of mess in the kitchen.

essential oils

Essential oils are the volatile oil component of a plant extracted through steam or hydro-distillation. They can also be produced by chemical extraction and then they tend to be called absolutes. Essential oils are very powerful medicines and should only be used externally unless you are directed by a professional medical herbalist, as they can easily be toxic if used in the wrong way. They can be added to ointments and creams to simply make them smell good or to add medicinal value to the preparation.

aromatic waters

Aromatic waters are also made through steam or hydro-distillation; the water-soluble part of the plant is extracted during the distillation process. Aromatic waters are safer to use internally than essential oils but are not readily available in Britain. They are light in flavour and contain no alcohol so are an ideal method of treating children and people who do not wish to use tinctures or teas.

enemas

Constipation is not the only reason for choosing this form of treatment. Enema therapy is getting more popular in this country with the development of colonic irrigation in posh clinics and health spas. It is a wonderful treatment for any bowel problem and for general detoxification of the whole body and bowel. Herbs can be used as warm infusions to create the enema fluid to soothe and calm irritated bowels or also to stimulate liver function and detoxify the body. Enema kits are commercially available.

douches

Douches are useful for treating infections within the vagina but I would not recommend using them frequently as they can alter the flora of the vagina and actually cause problems. To make a douche you make an infusion of appropriate herbs and use it as a wash. There are kits similar to an enema kit for douching.

baths

Herbal baths can be used as a tool to help the body and mind relax or to treat skin conditions. Essential oils, herb infusions, decoctions and infused oils can all be added to bath water for their therapeutic effects.

flower essences

Flower essences are not strictly considered herbal medicines as they do not have a chemical action on the body. They work on an energetic level, on the emotions and psyche. An individual may be physically affected as a result of using them but it is due to energetic rather than chemical activity.

the body systems

This chapter introduces each body system and acquaints you with many of the different things that can go wrong with them. I hope it will enable you to deepen your understanding of how and why things go wrong with each system and also how to fix them and keep them healthy.

Each body system section contains explanations of medical terms used to express the actions of the herbs required to treat various aspects of our health problems. These terms will be very useful, and I would encourage you to become familiar with them (see glossary on Page 158), mainly because most of the reference books on herbal medicine use this terminology even when written for the layman. Understanding these medical actions will guide your choice of herbal remedy for each situation you come across by helping you understand how to use the herbs to encourage better health and how to treat the root of any problem there may be with a particular system. For example, 'diaphoretic' is used to describe the action that a herb has and means it increases the body's ability to sweat, which may be useful in cases of fever where the body needs assistance in cooling down. An example of a diaphoretic herb is Elderflower.

Each individual body system is intrinsically linked to every other system so we need to consider the whole person in the treatment of any health problem. We therefore also show you how all the systems are linked to each other and when to consider treating other systems in conjunction with the main one.

At the end of each body system there is a quick reference section to give you ideas of herbs to use to treat common complaints linked to it. You can use these to get ideas for ways to safely use herbs to treat various disorders. For example a tea for rhinitis or a foot bath for flu. Once you have chosen the herb you want to use, refer to the 'the herbs' (see Page 61) section to find details of preparation and dosages to use and to 'how to make herbal medicines' (see Page 131) to find out how to make them.

the nervous system

It is within the nervous system that the connection between mind and body is most apparent. When anxiety affects us we have physical reactions such as heart palpitations, blushing, panic attacks and shortness of breath. When depression affects us physical symptoms can come in to play: a lack of energy, sleeping a lot, lack of motivation.

Sometimes it is the disease which causes the nervous system to become out of balance, for example flu causes depression in practically everyone although, luckily, it is usually short-lived. Other, chronic, diseases can also cause depression, long-term incapacity or a reduction in ability and function can be very frustrating and depressing.

Trauma can cause a feeling of panic and this emotion can drag on much longer than is necessary, causing a long term condition of anxiety and fear, even insomnia.

No matter what the cause behind the imbalance herbs can provide benefit in some way. There is an abundance of herbs for the nervous system and emotions and choosing the correct one is most important. For example, I have treated many people who have tried St. John's wort as an antidepressant without success, despite its reputation. This is because it was the wrong herb for their particular complaint. The basic rule in treating the nervous system with herbs is if the one you've chosen doesn't help within one month it isn't the right herb for you so try another one or consult a medical herbalist.

nervine tonics

Nervine tonics 'feed' and strengthen a depleted nervous system damaged, perhaps, by trauma, overwork and stress. The nervine tonic herbs help us to feel stronger, more able to cope with life and the stresses in our lives and they increase our mental and emotional stamina. The most popular nervine tonic amongst herbalists is Oats. This can be taken as a tincture, a tea, a capsule or you can just eat porridge (made the traditional way). Other tonics include Skullcap and Damiana. Damiana is also particularly good for nervousness around sexuality or for low self-esteem; it can help to raise a depleted libido and help you to feel good about yourself again.

nervine relaxants

Nervine relaxants help the mind and body to relax. They are used where stress and tension have built up or anxiety overwhelms and, in cases of insomnia, to aid sleep. Many nervine relaxants are also antispasmodic, working on the muscles to encourage physical relaxation too. Herbs with this nervine relaxant action include Wild Lettuce, Cramp bark, Lavender, Lime flower, Passionflower, Valerian and many more. When trying to choose which nervine relaxant is most appropriate for your needs, it is often helpful to look at their other actions and see which fits the specific needs best.

nervine stimulants

Perhaps the most fashionable herbal nervine stimulants are Coffee and Tea. They work to stimulate the nervous system and also have actions on the adrenal glands. They are very strong herbs and really should be treated as medicines: used as required not as a frequent beverage. Excessive or inappropriate use of these strong herbs can cause side effects from overstimulation of the nervous system and lead to anxiety, palpitations, decreased digestion, diarrhoea, constipation, arthritis, gastritis, depression and other imbalances. There are, however, gentler nervine stimulants which can be used to 'wake up' brain function, help memory, raise energy levels and aid concentration. Some good examples of these are Peppermint, Rosemary, and Sage; these are much gentler and can be drunk in moderation every day without side effects or risk of addiction.

antidepressants

It's been suggested that twenty-five per cent of the population is suffering from depression at any one time. Stress and the frustrations of life often lead us to feel low and depressed and these feelings can be alleviated by using antidepressant herbs. If you have a tendency to feel depressed they are also useful to take as a prophylactic. There are many antidepressant herbs and where the depression comes from and how it manifests itself is what guides a herbalist to choose the right one. For example, Orange flower is great for people who don't communicate when they get angry about something, they hold on to their anger becoming frustrated and eventually depressed. Orange flower helps them to express themselves more easily, cutting out the first step of their vicious cycle of depression. Whereas Rose is used to treat any type of depression associated with a broken heart or a loss of trust and Lemon balm soothes grief and allows us to let go and start to connect with life and being alive again.

anxiolytics

The anxiolytic herbs are mildly sedative like the nervine relaxants but they also have the specific action of relieving anxiety and any associated symptoms. Lime flower, for example, helps relieve anxiety which affects the heart causing palpitations and panic attacks. Valerian seems to take the edge off reality so that it isn't quite so scary and is useful for someone who experiences a lot of generalised fears. While Borage makes us more courageous and more able to face whatever life throws at us with inner strength.

herbs for the nervous system

anxiety

Affecting the stomach	Chamomile
Affecting the heart	Rose, Lime flower
Due to a lack of courage	Borage, Thyme
Due to trauma	Oats, Valerian

depression

Caused by trauma	Oats, Valerian, Rose
Caused by drugs, alcohol	Milk Thistle, Peppermint
Caused by negative thoughts	Passiflora, Lemon, Lemon balm, Peppermint
Caused by grief, loss	Rose, Lemon balm
Caused by anger	Peppermint, Chamomile, Lemon Balm

insomnia

Caused by over thinking	Valerian,
Waking early and not getting off to sleep again	Lime flower, Rose
Not getting off to sleep	Passiflora, Valerian, Lemon balm
Disturbed by dreams	Chamomile

tiredness and exhaustion

Caused by overwork	Liquorice, Borage
Associated with lack of motivation	Ginger
Associated with laziness and lack of exercise	Rosemary

headaches

Throbbing headache	Chamomile, Lavender
Hangover headache	Peppermint, Milk thistle
Sinus headache	Elderflower, Peppermint

migraine

Prevention	Feverfew, Lime flower
Associated nausea	Ginger, Peppermint

the respiratory system

We are not just what we eat – we are also what we breathe! Any problem with our breathing will affect the other parts of our body. If our breathing is inhibited this can cause the death or degeneration of tissues within the body. Our lungs are vital for our health and survival as they extract oxygen from the atmosphere which is essential for our cellular respiration, and eliminate carbon dioxide from our bodies, which in excess would be toxic. If our bodies are without oxygen for even a few minutes the brains cells die and cannot be replaced, causing impairment of the brain's function or, at worst, death.

As the lungs are organs of elimination they can be affected when the other organs of elimination, the skin, liver and kidneys, are in disharmony. If any of these are not working efficiently there is an increased load for the other organs to eliminate.

Circulation is also connected to the lungs' health as it is through the blood that the gases oxygen and carbon dioxide are transported around the body. Often when the heart is impaired the lungs suffer and, likewise, if the lungs are impaired the heart suffers. For example, in congestive heart failure where fluid can build up in the lung area and reduce the lungs' efficacy.

expectorants

Expectorants work by stimulating the nerve endings and muscles within the lungs causing them to expel more mucus from the lungs, increasing the cough response. They work well with mucolytics which break up sticky mucus so it is easier to expel. Some herbs are both mucolytic and expectorant like Thyme and Eucalyptus. Other herbs are more soothing and expectorant, useful for dry coughs, such as Marshmallow leaf.

antitussives

An antitussive is a respiratory relaxant and is of use when the muscles involved in breathing become tense or strained through excessive coughing or overexertion. They work to release tension and are helpful for any chest infection where there is lots of coughing causing a strained feeling in the chest. These herbs can, to some extent, suppress the cough response, which is especially useful in treating conditions like whooping cough. Good examples of antitussive herbs are Wild Cherry bark and Wild Lettuce.

demulcents

Demulcent herbs contain mucilage; this is a substance which feels slippery to touch and like mucus is very protective to our mucous membranes. It also acts to reduce inflammation and lubricate. Many herbs with this demulcent action also have other useful actions that can be used in treating lung complaints: Slippery elm and Marshmallow leaf, for example, are also both mild expectorants. Liquorice has steroidal-like activity and is highly anti-inflammatory.

anticatarrhal

These are herbs which help to reduce catarrh production. They can be used whether the catarrh is produced from allergy or infection. Nasal catarrh can also sometimes be due to other imbalances in the body. The anticatarrhal herbs will still be effective for symptomatic relief and the other problems need to be identified and addressed at the same time to create long-term change. Elderflower, Golden rod and Eyebright are probably the best anticatarrhals.

anti-inflammatory

Inflammation can occur in the respiratory system due to allergy, infection, systemic disease, smoking or just breathing bad air. This inflammation can be accompanied by other symptoms such as catarrh, cough, pain and mild shortness of breath. All these symptoms can be treated along with the inflammation to bring effective relief. Anti-inflammatory herbs specific to the lungs include Liquorice, Marshmallow leaf, Slippery elm and Plantain, which is especially useful in otitis (inflammation of the inner ear).

immune stimulants

Immune stimulants are called for wherever there is infection, a tendency to catch infections repeatedly or if low immunity has left you depleted, as with ME or chronic fatigue syndrome. Probably the most famous immune stimulant is Echinacea and it is a great one. However, it is an American import and we have herbs, like Elderflower or Elderberry, which are just as effective, native to this country. Traditionally Elderberries were collected in the autumn and made into a jam type substance called a 'rob'. A teaspoon of this rob would be taken once a day over the winter period and was said to prevent any occurrence of respiratory infection. Other herbs which have immune boosting properties include Ginger, Garlic and Peppermint.

antihistamine

Antihistamines for the respiratory system are useful in treating hayfever and allergic asthma. In the case of allergic asthma I would advise seeking help from a medical herbalist as there are certain restricted herbs which they can prescribe that are much more powerful than those generally available. There is, however, much you can do to reduce the histamine production by maintaining a good diet and using antihistamine herbs such as Nettle and Chamomile.

herbs for the respiratory system

colds & flu

Blocked nose	Peppermint, Elderflower
Runny nose	Golden rod, Eyebright
Fever	Lime flower, Elderflower, Peppermint
Aches	Bone set, Yarrow
Increase immune response	Echinacea, Elderflower, Lemon
Swollen glands	Calendula, Cleavers,
Sore throat	Sage, Thyme
Cough	Liquorice, Thyme, Marshmallow

hayfever

Itchy, sore eyes	Chamomile, Eyebright
Sore, itchy throat/sinuses	Plantain, Nettle, Marshmallow
Headaches	Elderflower, Peppermint
Funny taste in mouth	Peppermint, Eyebright, Golden rod

sinusitis

With runny nose	Golden rod, Eyebright, Plantain
With blocked nose	Elderflower, Peppermint, Plantain

earache

Associated with sore throat	Sage, Plantain, Echinacea
Associated with headache	Peppermint, Plantain, Elderflower

bronchitis & coughs

Associated with fever	Elderflower
Associated with tightness in chest	Cramp bark
Dry, non productive cough	Plantain, Marshmallow, Liquorice, Thyme
Productive cough	Lemon, Thyme,
Elecampane	
Associated with bad taste in mouth	Peppermint, Golden rod
Increase immune response	Echinacea, Elderflower, Lemon

the digestive system

Our overall health is very much dependent on the health of our digestive system and the quality of the food we put in it. If we are not getting the necessary nutrients to feed our cells and tissues then our health will eventually suffer.

The digestive system is approximately thirty-six feet long, starting with the mouth, moving through the oesophagus, the stomach and into the small intestines, where the pancreas, gall bladder and liver functions are involved with digestion and finally to the large intestine before the waste products are eliminated via the bowel. There are many organs and different regions of the intestines which can malfunction. In an ideal situation we can prevent disease by eating healthily, avoiding alcohol and cigarettes, having a balanced lifestyle, and having perfect genetics from our parents! However, in reality, we abuse our bodies in the name of pleasure: drinking and eating rich, unhealthy foods which irritate the stomach and clog up the bowel.

So, we are lucky that herbs provide us with a whole range of qualities which we can utilise to rebalance ourselves after a less than perfect lifestyle.

bitters

Bitters are pretty nasty-tasting herbs which stimulate the liver's production of bile and are often called cholagogues. Some are also called choleretics which means they stimulate the release of bile from the gall bladder. The bile is a useful digestive juice which aids digestion of fats and helps promote healthy bowel movements. The bitterest herbs include Wormwood and Gentian. Less bitter herbs include Dandelion root and Milk thistle seed.

hepatics

Hepatics are tonics for the liver function. They are also often bitter, cholagogues. Some hepatics also work to strengthen and protect the liver cells from toxins. Milk thistle is renowned for its ability to protect the liver from toxic chemicals and is very handy to have in the cupboard for a hangover. It helps to cleanse the liver of the toxic chemicals left behind following a night of drinking and repair some of the damage. Again, prevention is always better than cure and ideally Milk thistle should be taken a few hours before the party starts to protect the liver more effectively. Liquorice is another protective hepatic and is great to help constipation, which is often associated with poor liver function.

sialogogues

These are herbs which increase saliva production. Saliva contains a digestive enzyme called amylase which breaks down carbohydrates into smaller compounds which can then be digested in the stomach. This is why chewing food is important as this first step in digestion is necessary to aid the stomach's processes. If you don't chew well enough, or if you have insufficient saliva, this can cause bloating and pain as the stomach simply cannot digest what it has been given. Sialogogues include bitters and other herbs such as Peppermint, Fennel, Calendula and Liquorice.

laxatives and evacuants

Laxatives and evacuants can work in several ways, all with the same aim: to make you poo! Some laxatives work to increase the flow of digestive juices, particularly bile, to help the digestion process produce a firm but moist stool, easy to pass, with no straining or discomfort. Such herbs include the bitters and others such as Liquorice, Peppermint, and Fennel.

The evacuants are less gentle; they stimulate bowel function by forcing the bowel to spasm and mimic the natural process of peristalsis (a wave of muscular contraction which moves through the whole digestive tract). They can, unfortunately, be physically addictive and, if taken long term, reduce the ability of the bowel to move itself. With this in mind the strong evacuants should only be used when essential. Perhaps a healthier option is to use a liquid enema, although this is not to everyone's taste! Examples of evacuant herbs are senna, rhubarb root (Rheum palmatum not the garden variety), Cascara sagrada, Aloe and Buckthorn. A side effect of using these herbs can be painful cramps so I would advise using them with an antispasmodic to reduce this reaction.

antiemetics

These are herbs which reduce nausea and prevent vomiting. Whether it is caused by a viral infection, travel sickness or pregnancy, Ginger is the best one to try. The powder, in capsules, seems to work best as drying the herbs causes a change in the chemistry making its action even stronger. Other useful antiemetics include Peppermint, Meadowsweet and Lemon Balm.

anthelmintics

These are herbs which work to eliminate parasitic worms from the intestines. Wormwood is one good example and it's easy to remember what it does with a name like that! There are other herbs that have been used traditionally as enemas for this problem: Garlic is one and Quassia bark chips another. These treatments work best in conjunction with fasting but do consult an experienced herbalist to support the procedures if they are new to you. Fasting can be dangerous for some individuals and should not be done without professional guidance.

demulcents

Demulcents are used in the treatment of the lungs and the urinary system as well as the digestive system. They are mucilaginous herbs which produce a substance that helps to coat and protect mucous membranes whilst also reducing inflammation. The herb Marshmallow is used for all three systems: the leaf is more specific for the bladder and lungs and the root for the digestive system. Demulcents can also help to relieve constipation where the stools are dry and the stomach and intestines are irritable.

carminatives

Carminative herbs help the digestive system to release wind gently and appropriately. They relax the muscles which may be cramping up around the gas and also increase gentle peristalsis enabling the wind to move through and out of the bowel. They also help the digestive function so that less wind is produced in the first place, thereby helping to reduce the distension, bloating and pain experienced in association with wind. There are many carminative herbs, all have essential oil components and are highly aromatic. They include Peppermint, Cardamom, Caraway, Fennel, Ginger, Chamomile, Angelica and Thyme.

astringents

Astringent herbs help to condense tissue by causing a contraction in individual cell walls. This action is helpful in the treatment of digestive disorders where there may be a leaky gut wall causing allergies and sensitivities to food. Other causes of inflammation in the bowel can also cause leaky gut problems and astringents can be used in all these cases from general diarrhoea caused by a viral infection to irritable bowel syndrome and diverticulas.

antispasmodics

Cramps and colicky pains in the gut can have underlying causes which need to be identified: perhaps bad diet, poor digestive function or gastritis. These conditions need specific treatment and antispasmodics can be a part of it. The antispasmodic herbs include Peppermint, Cramp bark, Chamomile and Valerian.

antimicrobials

Infections within the digestive system are very common, especially where immunity is low, diet is bad and life is stressful. Children seem particularly prone to virus-induced gastritis causing diarrhoea and vomiting and antimicrobials can be of great benefit especially when used with antiemetics, diaphoretics and immune boosting herbs. The best antimicrobials specific for the digestive system are Myrrh, Echinacea, Peppermint, Thyme and Wormwood. Candida is another pathogen which has been in the limelight over the last few years and if you suspect you have Candida problems the herbs listed above are also antifungal and could be used to clear a systemic Candida infection.

herbs for the digestive system

constipation

Dry stools	Marshmallow, Slippery elm
Irritable bowel syndrome	Marshmallow
	Chamomile, Peppermint
Sluggish digestion	Rhubarb, Milk thistle, Dandelion root

diarrhoea

Due to food intolerance	Slippery elm, Chamomile
Associated with nausea	Peppermint, Chamomile

loss of appetite

Due to worry, anxiety	Valerian, Chamomile
Associated with anorexia	Wormwood
Associated with bloating	Peppermint, Fennel

indigestion

Associated with heartburn	Slippery elm, Marshmallow
Associated with bloating	Fennel, Cardamom Peppermint
Associated with cramps	Cramp bark, Peppermint, Chamomile

gastritis

Due to food intolerance	Slippery elm, Chamomile
Associated with cramps	Cramp bark, Peppermint, Chamomile
Associated with diarrhoea	Raspberry leaf, Lemon balm

haemorrhoids

Active bleeding piles	Yarrow, Horse chestnut
Inactive not bleeding piles	Hawthorn, Yarrow, Horse chestnut
Due to food intolerance	Slippery elm, Chamomile
Associated with cramps	Cramp bark, Peppermint,
Associated with diarrhoea	Raspberry leaf, Lemon balm
Associated with constipation	Slippery elm, Marshmallow

gingivitis

Associated with bleeding gums	Myrrh, Calendula, Yarrow
Associated with abscess	Echinacea, Calendula, Myrrh

the circulatory system

The circulation, like the nervous system, is connected to every part of us and therefore affects every part of us. It is a transport system for food and oxygen to feed our tissues and also a carrier for toxins which need to be eliminated via the kidneys, liver, lungs and skin. It is also closely connected to our lymphatic system which works mainly to cleanse our bodies of waste products excreted by cells and tissues.

The circulatory system includes the heart, arteries, arterioles, veins and capillaries. Any of these parts may be affected in their own right or need treatment due to their connection to organs or tissues.

Prevention is always easier than cure and diet, lifestyle and exercise all play an important part in the health of our circulation. Lifestyle factors which are unhelpful to this system's health are alcohol, fat, smoking, stress, lack of exercise and salt. Regular exercise to work the heart and circulation is a sure way to keep the blood moving and helping it to be cleansed as it is pushed through the liver, lungs and kidneys that bit faster. Stress and emotional tensions really do have a connection to our heart function, this is why we use the term broken-hearted. Herbs can be used to alleviate symptoms of stress and emotional upset whilst other therapies, for example counselling, art therapy, hypnotherapy, shamanic healing, can be employed if the herbs are not enough to change the negative pattern on their own.

heart tonics

Probably the best herb for the heart and circulation in general is Hawthorn. The flowers or berries feed the heart, strengthening it and toning the muscle. It is one of the few herbs which I would recommend people take on a longer-term basis if there is any genetic link to heart failure or if they have suffered any heart problems in the past. However, it can interact with some heart medications by making those medications more effective, so less is required. This can be viewed as a positive or negative but if you are on heart medication do not use this herb without professional advice first. Regular check-ups should also be done to ensure the medications are at the correct level for your needs and do not produce unwanted side effects. Motherwort is also considered a heart tonic as it has a powerful nervine effect which calms the emotions affecting the heart.

There are some stronger heart tonics available from qualified herbalists for the treatment of heart failure and angina. They are safe but restricted, for example, Lily of the Valley. Digitalis from the foxglove was also once used by herbalists but is now restricted to prescription by medical doctors only as it can cause dangerous side effects in excessive doses.

circulatory tonics

General circulation can become impaired causing bruising, haemorrhoids, varicose veins, chilblains and can also be inadequate in supplying tissues, causing degeneration of other tissues or organ function as a result. Hawthorn is one of the best herbs as a normaliser of circulation and heart function. Other herbs help to increase the integrity of cell walls within the capillaries to prevent bruising, or bleeding such as Yarrow and Horse chestnut. Horse chestnut is highly astringent to the veins and can reduce problems with piles and varicose veins. Ginger, Cayenne and Yarrow are peripheral circulatory stimulants; they help the blood to flow to the extremities of the body and to the tissues which have limited circulation such as joints, tendons, ligaments, and hands, fingers, toes and feet. This can be beneficial for people who feel cold a lot of the time. There are also herbs which are considered cooling to the blood which aid peripheral circulation such as Gingko and Lime flower.

diuretics

When the heart is weak and failing to circulate the blood efficiently water can build up in the body causing oedema in the legs or around the lungs. Heart tonics are often called for in this event. However, diuretics can help to reduce the strain on the heart. Dandelion is especially useful due to its high potassium content, helping to maintain the potassium balance within the body. Other useful diuretic herbs for relief of circulatory problems include Yarrow and Lime flower.

nervines

Where stress is affecting the heart or causing hypertension, relaxing nervines are called for. Motherwort has a particular affinity for the heart whilst being calming. Rose is very effective where there is any form of heartbreak or anger causing emotional upset. Lime flower helps to relax the anxious person who may also suffer from palpitations. Skullcap and Valerian are great for people who just can't stop worrying about everything.

hypotensives

Hypotensives can work by increasing peripheral circulation or decreasing the stress response. So here we need to look for certain types of circulatory tonic and also relaxing nervines. A blend of the two is usually best. Lime flower and Yarrow are great herbs for this as they do both, acting as a mild nervine and a peripheral circulation stimulant.

herbs for the circulatory system

high blood pressure

Due to stress, anxiety	Valerian, Passionflower
Associated with heart palpitations	Lime flower, Rose
Associated with high cholesterol	Garlic, Hawthorn berry, Lime flower
Associated with lack of exercise	Cramp bark, Gingko
Associated with oedema	Dandelion leaf, Yarrow

low blood pressure

Associated with feeling cold	Ginger, Cinnamon
Associated with poor appetite or digestion	Cardamom, Cinnamon, Wormwood, Dandelion root, Milk thistle
Associated with dizziness	Rosemary
Associated with stress	Oat straw, Hawthorn

poor circulation

Associated with cold hands and feet	Ginger, Gingko, Chilli/ Cayenne
Associated with cold back	Ginger, Rosemary, Juniper berry
Chilblains	Ginger, Hawthorn berry

varicose veins

All types	Horse chestnut, Yarrow, Ginkgo

maintaining a healthy heart

Strengthening the heart	Hawthorn, Motherwort
When anxiety affects the heart	Lime flower, Lemon balm

the genitourinary system

These two systems are situated in the same region of the body and some of the anatomy is shared. The two systems have very different functions and, most of the time, require different actions from different herbs. Occasionally the systems are linked by disease, for example prostatitis, and during pregnancy where there is a need to urinate frequently and, sometimes, recurrent cystitis.

The urinary system's main function is to eliminate toxins. The kidneys clean and filter the blood, removing the toxins and sending them on to the bladder for storage until there is enough to warrant urination. The kidneys are also involved in the regulation of blood pressure.

The gynaecological system is mainly concerned with procreation and its functioning revolves around this. There are many ailments commonly associated with both the female and the male reproductive organs. Many of the herbs traditionally thought of as 'female' herbs can also be used to tonify the male reproductive system as they increase circulation to the area, cleansing and nourishing it and helping to sustain healthy functioning.

antispasmodics

Antispasmodics can be of use to women during menstruation if they suffer from cramping period pains. The more powerful antispasmodics associated with the genitourinary system can also be used to relieve the cramping which comes with passing kidney stones (gravel).

uterine tonics

The uterine tonics strengthen and tone the tissues and function of the reproductive organs. These herbs are also useful tonics for the male reproductive system but were not used widely for this purpose until recently. Raspberry leaf has a reputation for enabling a speedy birth process free of pain and complications. It can be drunk safely from the second trimester of the pregnancy all the way through to labour and the birth itself. It is useful for treating any problem associated with the uterine area such as endometriosis, irregular periods, scanty bleeding, heavy bleeding, and thrush. Other uterine tonics include *Mitchella repens* and Motherwort.

emmenagogues

These are herbs which encourage a delayed period and help to regulate periods. Some emmenagogues are thought to work as tonics and others are thought to irritate the system causing it to get rid of its contents and have been used as abortificants in the past. These herbs should be avoided during pregnancy and are not a safe (or legal) way to produce an abortion. The irritating emmenagogues include Pennyroyal and Blue cohosh. Gentler emmenagogues include Motherwort, Wormwood and Yarrow.

menstrual regulators

Whether periods are too frequent or too far between, menstrual regulators will help the cycle to normalise. Some work by acting on the hormonal system, regulating and balancing the hormones which in turn regulate the menstrual cycle. These include Vitex agnus castus and Black cohosh. Others act as tonics to the reproductive system in general such as Sage, Raspberry leaf and Yarrow.

alteratives

As the lower abdomen is prone to congestion and toxicity, and this congestion automatically affects the organs of the genitourinary system, alteratives can often be of benefit when treating any condition in the area. They help to cleanse and improve the health of all the tissues. Alteratives specifically useful for this area include Calendula, Cleavers, Echinacea and Sage. Calendula and Sage also have a reputation for healing scar tissue in the uterine area and, as a result, possibly increase the level of fertility in women who have suffered chlamydia and have scar damage to the fallopian tubes.

nervines

Nervines are effective for the genitourinary system in several ways. They can act to enhance libido, for example Damiana and

Rose and they can bring relief from symptoms of pre-menstrual tension, for example Valerian and *Anemone pulsatilla*. They can also be of benefit as analgesics when there is any pain from periods, kidney stones (gravel) and other problems. The strongest nervines are restricted to prescription by herbalists as they can have side effects at inappropriate doses.

antiseptics

Where there is infection within the genitourinary system, antiseptics are called for. They can be taken internally, blended with an immune-boosting herb and a soothing demulcent herb. They can also be used externally as a wash, a herbal aromatic water spray, in the bath or as a sitz bath. Useful herbs for external use include Lavender, Chamomile, Calendula, Rose, Comfrey and for itching use Chickweed. Herbs such as Golden rod, Elderflower and Calendula can be used internally.

demulcents

Demulcents produce a soothing effect on the mucous membranes where infection, friction or allergy has irritated them. Useful demulcent herbs include Marshmallow and Cornsilk. Comfrey is a demulcent and has a particularly cooling and soothing effect when used in a sitz bath.

diuretics

Diuretics increase the urine output from the kidneys. They can be useful when there is retention of fluid in the body or when you need to flush out an infection in the urinary system. Dandelion leaf is a very effective and safe diuretic to use as it has a high level of potassium and prevents the loss of this mineral from the blood, unlike some other diuretics. Many other herbs also have diuretic properties such as Elderflower and Cleavers.

herbs for the genitourinary system

cystitis & urethritis

Associated with fever	Elderflower, Golden rod, Echinacea
Painful urination	Marshmallow leaf, Cornsilk
Long history of symptoms	Uva ursi, Cranberry, Nettle
Associated with incontinence	Horsetail, Cornsilk

water retention

Associated with poor circulation	Yarrow, Dandelion leaf
Associated with weak kidney function	Cornsilk, Dandelion leaf

pre-menstrual tension

Associated with anger	Rose, Chamomile, Lavender
Associated with tearfulness	Pasque flower, Valerian
Associated with bloating	Yarrow, Cornsilk

irregular periods

Lack of periods	Raspberry leaf, Cardamom
Scanty bleeding	*Angelica sinensis*, Rosemary
Excessive bleeding	Yarrow, Ladies mantle
Painful periods	Cramp bark, Raspberry leaf, Valerian
Swollen breasts	Calendula, Red clover

menopausal problems

Anxiety, palpitations	Motherwort, Limeflower, Rose
Hot flushes, night sweats	Sage, Red clover, Liquorice
Tiredness, lethargy	Siberian ginseng, Rosemary, Borage
Vaginal dryness	Comfrey, Evening primrose

low sex drive

Associated with tiredness, stress	Siberian ginseng, Liquorice, Damiana
Feeling unattractive	Jasmine flowers, Rose, Damiana

thrush

Associated with an itchy rash	Chickweed, Marigold
Associated with inflammation	Lavender, Marigold, Rose
Associated with dryness	Comfrey, Rose
Associated with a discharge	Lady's mantle, White dead nettle
Associated with systemic symptoms	Marigold, Echinacea, Wormwood

the musculoskeletal system

The health of the musculoskeletal system is essential to enable us to sit, stand and move freely and without pain. It takes a lot of wear and tear over the years and we can prevent a lot of the disorders that can occur simply by having a good diet and getting beneficial exercise. Where there are structural misalignments it is best to seek the help of a good, registered osteopath who can manipulate the structure directly and teach you how to take better care of yourself so the problem doesn't reoccur. Studying Alexander technique can help if the problem is linked to posture.

Sometimes we have a genetic disposition to certain types of disease. This does not mean we have to suffer them; it means we need to adjust our lifestyle and diet to suit our health needs and reduce the degree to we which we are affected by our hereditary health problems.

Musculoskeletal problems have links with other systems in the body: namely the circulatory, lymphatic, digestive and urinary systems. The circulatory and lymphatic systems help to feed the tissues, cleansing and detoxifying them, preventing degeneration and toxic build-up. The digestive system is also linked as it is responsible for assimilation of food, absorbing the nutrients from our food for the nourishment of all of the body's tissues. It also has an eliminatory function. The urinary system is responsible for eliminating some of the toxins which typically build up in arthritic conditions and can benefit from support when this occurs.

antirheumatics

An antirheumatic herb can have one or more actions: it could aid elimination, reduce inflammation, increase circulation and relieve pain. Such herbs include Black cohosh, Bogbean, Celery, Cayenne, Dandelion, Ginger, Juniper, Nettle, Mustard, Wormwood and Yarrow.

alteratives

Alteratives cleanse and nourish a toxic area of tissue. Rheumatism and arthritis are caused by toxic build-up in joints and tissues so alteratives are always called for in their treatment. Herbs with this action specific to the musculoskeletal system include Celery, Black cohosh, Dandelion, Burdock, Juniper and Nettle.

anti-inflammatories

Inflammation is involved in many musculoskeletal problems and is the cause of most pain. Herbs which reduce inflammation do not simply suppress the problem: they help the body to overcome it. Meadowsweet is a perfect example as it helps to eliminate the waste and toxins which have built up and also contains salicylic acid which has an aspirin-like action reducing inflammation and pain. Other anti-inflammatory herbs specific for this system include Celery, White willow, Black willow, White poplar, Devil's Claw and Wild Yam.

antispasmodics

Antispasmodics can be used when there has been a strain or sprain in any muscle of the body and which is inflamed and cramping. The herbs can be used internally to good effect and by application to the affected area by using a topical cream, ointment, oil or compress. Essential oils are good for this external application as they are such small chemicals they are able to get through the skin very quickly and bring fast relief. Useful essential oils include Lavender, Clary sage, Chamomile or Sweet Marjoram and infused St. John's wort oil is the most effective base oil to use as a carrier massage oil. Herbs which can be taken internally or applied externally include Cramp Bark, Valerian, Chamomile and Rosemary.

rubefacients

Rubefacients are applied to the skin, rather than taken internally. They heat the area, increasing circulation, relieving congestion and reducing inflammation. They are very strong and should not be used on broken or damaged skin. Some rubefacients appear to have a cooling action on the tissues, useful where the joint feels hot or is worse for heat. These include Peppermint oil and Lemon-scented Eucalyptus oil. Other rubefacients are warming like Cayenne, Rosemary, Mustard and Ginger.

diuretics

Diuretics that encourage the body to eliminate toxins and the products of inflammation are essential in treating arthritis and rheumatism. It is the kidneys which eliminate most of the toxins associated with these problems and sometimes they need a little support when there is a significant build up. Herbs such as Celery and Cleavers are most useful and general tonics for the kidneys such as Nettle and Juniper are also worth considering.

circulatory stimulants

Circulatory stimulants are used primarily to aid the elimination of toxins and secondly to encourage nutrition into any damaged area to aid healing. The herbs used for this purpose are not stimulating the heart function but aiding peripheral circulation through the capillaries which feed into the affected tissues. The herbs which help peripheral circulation include Ginger, Cayenne, Rosemary and Gingko.

pain relievers

Of course the best way to relieve the pain on a long term basis is to remove the cause but while you do this the analgesic herbs can help. Some herbs which can have an analgesic effect include White willow, Meadowsweet and Valerian.

digestive tonics

People with musculoskeletal problems often also have poor digestion and elimination. The digestive process has to work properly so that vital nutrients are fed into the delicate tissues which make up our bones, and elimination of toxins is also vital so they do not cause congestion and inflammation. So, by working on the digestion we can improve the health of the musculoskeletal system. Some of the digestive tonics are especially good for this purpose including Devils claw, Dandelion root, Gentian, Wormwood and Yarrow.

herbs for the musculoskeletal system

inflammation affecting the skeletal system

Osteoarthritis, internal use	Celery seed, Devil's claw, Meadowsweet
If worse when cold	Ginger, Juniper
If worse when hot	*Eucalyptus citriodora* oil
Gout	Celery seed, Yarrow, Dandelion root
Associated with insomnia	Valerian, Passion flower

backache

Associated with muscle spasm	Cramp bark, Ginger
Lower back ache which feels cold	Juniper, Ginger

sciatica

External oil	St. Johns wort
Internal herbs	St. Johns wort, Calendula
Associated with constipation	Rhubarb root

sprains

Affecting any area	Arnica ointment, Daisy ointment, Hot bath with Rosemary, Everlasting essential oil

the skin

The skin has many functions; it protects from infection by micro-organisms and acts as an organ of elimination for approximately twenty-five per cent of the body's waste products. If the skin's eliminatory function becomes impaired this can put extra strain on the other eliminatory organs within the body: namely the kidneys, liver and lungs. In the same way, if any of these organs are not functioning correctly the skin will have to work extra hard and may show signs and symptoms of disease.

The skin also has a close association with the nervous system; it is rich with sensory nerve endings which allow us to feel and be in contact with our environment. Skin can also show signs of emotional or nervous disorders and, if the skin is diseased, this affects how we feel within ourselves. From blushing to eczema, the skin is often a reflection of the internal state of being.

vulneraries

A vulnerary herb is one which helps to heal damage to the skin's surface. There are several ways a herb can work to heal the skin more quickly. Comfrey, for example, actually speeds up cell regeneration: increasing the rate of mitosis (cell division) so that the repaired tissue heals much faster. Comfrey also encourages the regeneration of normal tissue, instead of scar tissue, making it a very attractive herb to use post-operatively once the stitches are out. Comfrey was traditionally called Knitbone because its fast action was used to heal bone tissue following breaks and fractures.

The other way vulneraries work is to astringe the tissue, to tighten them, which helps to stop bleeding and draw the edges of the tissue together. A prime example of this is Yarrow: also known as Nosebleed due to its ability to arrest bleeding.

Some herbs are able to provide a protective barrier across a wound, preventing infection while healing occurs. Myrrh is one such herb; it is also highly anti-microbial and is very useful for the first aid box, particularly in a liquid form such as a tincture or essential oil.

alteratives

Alteratives can be thought of as cleansing herbs. They alter the condition of a tissue, detoxifying polluted areas and helping to restore proper healthy functioning. The herbs that are termed alterative can be specific to certain tissues or organs or they can be general detoxifiers for the whole body. Dandelion root works to clear the liver, Dandelion leaf clears the kidneys, Echinacea cleans the blood, Blue flag cleans the skin and Cleavers cleanses the lymphatic system. Alteratives are usually of great benefit when treating skin complaints as the condition will usually be associated with poor elimination via one organ or another. Psoriasis is linked to the liver and blood, eczema to the lungs and kidneys. Acne is also associated with hormones but, as the liver is the organ which eliminates excess hormones, the hormone imbalance can be treated by using alteratives to increase the liver function.

antimicrobials

Anti-microbials are called for when pathogens have invaded the skin and caused a problem. They can work directly on the pathogen or they work to increase the immune response so the body fights harder. Thyme is a very powerful, direct anti-microbial and can be used to treat infections from fungi, bacteria and viruses. Echinacea however, works to increase the immune response.

antihistamine

Antihistamine herbs help to reduce the inflammatory response associated with a histamine reaction. These reactions occur due to an external stimulus, such as a mosquito bite, or an internal imbalance, such as eczema or an allergic reaction like hayfever or urticaria. Whatever the cause, these herbs help to reduce the inflammation, itching and pain caused by excess histamine in the body. Some herbs, such as Chickweed, are best used externally. Chickweed can reduce itching in many cases where nothing else seems to work. Even the itching caused by some orthodox drugs is relieved when Chickweed ointment is applied. Nettle leaf is used internally to treat all sorts of histamine reactions from hayfever to eczema.

herbs for the skin

acne
Associated with hormonal imbalance	Raspberry leaf, Nettle root
Associated with poor diet	Cleavers, Echinacea
External application	Marigold, Echinacea

boils
Any boil	Marigold, Echinacea, Yarrow
External application	Marigold, Echinacea, Marshmallow leaf poultice

fungal infections
Best treated externally if acute	Palmarosa or Tea tree essential oil
If chronic, treat internally also	Echinacea, Marigold

warts and verrucae
All types	Lemon essential oil, neat, Thuja tincture

bruises
On closed skin	Arnica or daisy ointment
On broken skin	Marigold, Comfrey

cuts and grazes
To stop bleeding	Yarrow, Myrrh
To heal skin	Marigold, Comfrey
To remove grit in a graze	Honey plasters
To prevent infection	Tea tree essential oil, honey, Marigold

burns
Cool down ASAP!	
To heal skin	Lavender, Marigold, Comfrey
To prevent infection	Lavender, Marigold

eczema
Weeping eczema	Bathe with oak bark infusion
Dry eczema	Chamomile, Nettle, Red clover
Itchy eczema	Chickweed, Nettle, Chamomile

the herbs

This chapter contains forty-four herb monographs describing common herbs you can grow, collect from the wild or buy in local shops. There are over two thousand herbs used in European herbal medicine, so the list is far from complete. It is, however, more than enough for you to be able to begin your journey and be really effective in your treatments. By using an exclusive range of herbs, and those readily available to you, you can get to know this selection of herbs really well and understand how best to use them to treat a whole realm of common complaints and conditions. There is just one herb included which is a little more difficult to find in Europe as it is harvested from the deserts of Africa. It is Myrrh and, once as precious as Gold, its properties are so unique and powerfully therapeutic it had to be included. I find Myrrh constantly useful in the treatment of so many ailments and I think it is worth the extra effort needed to source it from more specialist shops.

When you are collecting herbs from the wild it is really important that you collect exactly what you mean to, so I suggest you always use a reliable field guide. The one I recommend is *The Wild Flower Key: A Guide to Plant Identification in the Field, with and Without Flowers* by Francis Rose (see Page 166 for full details).

angelica

Angelica archangelica

parts used
Roots, leaves and seeds for medicinal use and the stem and seeds in flavouring and sweets or liqueurs.

collection
The roots are collected in the autumn after the first year of growth and will benefit from being cut into smaller sections to help aid drying. The stem and leaves can be collected earlier in the year, in June. The seed should be collected in the autumn of the second year once the plant has had a chance to fully mature.

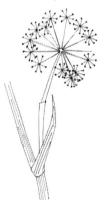

cultivation
This plant is easy to grow from fresh seed and the seed should be sown as soon as it ripens, between August and September. It can also be multiplied by root division. Angelica takes two years to mature and plants should be grown one metre apart in their second year.

constituents
Veleric acid, angelic acid, sugar, bitter principle, angelicin. The essential oil from the root also contains terpenes including terebangelene. The oil from the seeds contains methis, methyl-ethylacetic acid and hydroxymyristic acid.

actions
The roots, stalks and the leaves of this plant all have carminative, stomachic, warming and mildly diaphoretic properties. It is anti-fungal, expectorant, an antispasmodic, emmenagogue and diuretic.

indications
gastrointestinal system
It is used for weak digestion and flatulence, and will warm and tone the stomach so that food is digested more effectively.

respiratory system
It is traditionally used as an expectorant and warming diaphoretic for chest problems such as bronchitis, pleurisy, colic and for coughs and colds.

genitourinary system
A mild emmenagogue.

musculoskeletal system
Angelica has a reputation for relieving gout and rheumatism. This is probably due to its warming digestive and diaphoretic actions so that it helps to increase absorption of nutrients to the body whilst simultaneously having a mildly detoxifying action.

immune system
It acts as a general tonic for anyone who is debilitated by illness, exhaustion or stress and suffering from a cold or cold-like symptoms with poor digestion.

contraindications
Pregnancy and diabetes.

preparations and dosage
tea use 1–2 teaspoons per cup, infuse for 10 minutes and drink three times daily. The root is usually used for tea but leaf and seed can also be used.

tincture 1 part herb to 5 parts 45% alcohol, infuse for 4 days, macerate daily. Take 5ml in water three times daily.

balsam a product made by macerating the root in alcohol, then evaporating the alcohol off so the residue can be collected. This is a complex technique and balsams are commercially available (See Page 163).

combinations
For a digestive tonic, mix with a nourishing demulcent herb like Marshmallow root and a cooling balancing herb like Chamomile. To use as part of a respiratory blend to treat a chesty cough, add a demulcent herb like Marshmallow, using the leaf, and a mucolytic herb such as Thyme.

basil

Ocimum basilicum

parts used
Leaves.

collection
Collect when the plant has matured but before it dies back in the autumn.

cultivation

Seeds are sown annually. They can be sown indoors all year round but need plenty of warmth and sun to flourish. They can be sown out doors in a warm sheltered sunny spot from the last week of April and prefer a fairly rich soil. Using a hot bed will increase your success.

constituents

The essential oil contains: monoterpenols including linalool, ethers 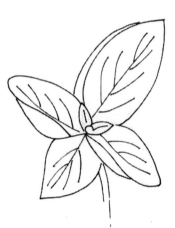 including methyl chavicol, methyl eugenol, phenols including eugenol, oxides including 1,8 cineole, sesquiterpenes including germacrene D, elemene, α-bergamotene, β-caryophyllene, monoterpenes including ocimene, α and β-pinene, esters including bornyl acetate and many other trace compounds.

actions

The essential oil is anticatarrhal, antidepressive, antifungal, antiseptic, antispasmodic, carminative, cephalic, diaphoretic, digestive stimulant, emmenagogue, expectorant, galactogogue, nervine, restorative, tonic.

indications

digestive system

Helpful for treating poor digestive function and symptoms including irritable bowel syndrome (IBS), flatulence, bloating and associated pain. As an antispasmodic it can also relieve the cramping pains associated with IBS and wind.

respiratory system

Traditionally used in Ayurvedic medicine as a treatment for coughs, bronchitis, colds and asthma to encourage expectoration of phlegm from the lungs.

nervous system

The 'cephalic' action of Basil means that it increases blood circulation to the head and is effective in improving memory and concentration – a good herb to use when studying. Basil is also calming and antidepressive in nature and can alternatively be used to treat insomnia.

contraindications

The essential oil should not be used on children under two years and is to be avoided by people with damaged or hypersensitive skin. It should be diluted to 2% maximum in massage preparations. The herb itself is safest to use for self-treatment.

preparations and dosage

tea use 1–2 teaspoons per cup, infuse for 10 minutes and drink three times daily.

tincture 1 part herb to 5 parts 45% alcohol, infuse for four days, macerate daily. Take 5ml in water three times daily.

combinations

In my opinion this herb is best simply added to salads as a nerve strengthener and general cephalic to aid memory and other mental functions.

bay laurel

Laurus nobolis

parts used

Leaves, fruit.

collection

A small evergreen tree, it has leaves all year round ready to collect.

cultivation

It grows well under the shade of other trees and can be kept clipped as a very ornamental, evergreen shrub. You often see them in garden centres clipped into cute lollipop shapes.

constituents

The essential oil distilled from the leaves and contains: oxides including 1,8 cineole, terpenes including α & β-pinene, β-sabinene, β-elemene, β-caryophyllene, alcohols including linalol, α-terpineol & terpineol-4, esters including terpenyl acetate, phenols including eugenol; methyl-ether, methyl-ether and many other trace compounds.

actions
Antibacterial, anticatarrhal, antifungal, neurotonic anti-infectious, antispasmodic, antirheumatic, carminative, digestive tonic, mild diuretic, expectorant,.

indications
digestive system
A general tonic for the digestive system which promotes healthy digestion and elimination from the bowel. It alleviates bloating and spasmodic pains.

musculoskeletal system
A powerful antispasmodic and antirheumatic oil which alleviates aches, pains and general fatigue in the muscles.

respiratory system
A powerful herb for this system, it clears phlegm from the lungs and catarrh from the sinuses. It can be used to treat bronchitis, colds, flu, laryngitis and sinusitis.

nervous system
The essential oil is a tonic for the nervous system. It stimulates circulation to the head and can be used to treat poor memory and concentration. Its general tonic action stimulates mind and body encouraging us to be bold and self-confident.

contraindications
This essential oil should not be used on children under two years or people with sensitive or damaged skin, and should be used at a maximum dilution of 2%.

preparations and dosage
essential oil used in a bath, add just 4 drops for effect.
Bay Laurel is generally only used as a food flavouring herb now and not taken internally. It is actually very powerful for something we are used to adding to our food. The berries were traditionally used in herbal medicine for their toxic effects and this should never be tried without the advice of a professional herbalist.

combinations
It can be used to flavour food, for example add 2 bay leaves when preparing a litre of stock or soup. Or the fresh leaves can be used in a bath, which gives a very stimulating and generally tonic bath for the whole body and mind.

borage

Borago officinalis

parts used
Dried leaves and flowers.

collection
The leaves and flowers are collected just as the plant is coming into flower in early summer. Collect on a dry day and strip off individual leaves and flowers so they can dry more quickly.

cultivation
Very easy to grow from seed. Sow into pots or straight into the soil in April, and place in a sunny position for best results in well drained and rich soil.

constituents
Pyrrolizadine alkaloids, choline, saponins, tannins, mucilage, essential oil.

actions
Adrenal gland restorative, galactagogue, demulcent, emollient, diuretic, antidepressive, diaphoretic, expectorant, general tonic, anti-inflammatory.

indications
endocrine system
Borage works as a restorative to the adrenal cortex and can therefore be used to revive its function after medical treatment involving steroids or cortisone. As stress also depletes this gland it is a very good herb for general tiredness, depression and nervous exhaustion.

immune system
As a diaphoretic it can be used to reduce fevers, has a reputation as an expectorant and anti-inflammatory and can be helpful in inflammatory respiratory conditions like pleurisy.

contraindications
None known.

preparations and dosage
tea use 1–2 teaspoons per cup, infuse for 10 minutes and drink three times daily.
tincture 1 part herb to 5 parts 45% alcohol, infuse for four days, macerate daily. Take 5ml in water three times daily.

combinations
To treat feverish respiratory infections use it with Lime flower, Elderflower and Echinacea. As a remedy for depression it works well with Rose and Peppermint.

celery

Apium graveolens

parts used
Seeds.

collection
The seeds should be collected when ripe in the autumn.

cultivation
This plant has a reputation for being a little difficult to grow and seedlings need to be started indoors. Start by sowing the seeds in pots and, when they have germinated and are large enough to thin, remove most of them leaving just two or three. Eventually remove all but the largest plant in each pot. Transplant outdoors after the last frost spacing the plants 30cms apart, in rows 60-75cm apart. They like a lot of water too so need consistent attention.

constituents
The plant contains 2–3% essential oil, apiol, coumarins, minerals iron, phosphorous, potassium, sodium.

actions
Alkaline reaction on the blood, anti-rheumatic, urinary antiseptic, diuretic, antispasmodic, carminative, tonic digestive, galactagogue, assists elimination of uric acid, Anti-gout, anti-inflammatory, hypotensor, aphrodisiac.

indications
musculoskeletal system
Celery seed's main use is in the treatment of arthritis and gout where there is a build-up of uric acid crystals in the joints and an associated problem with excretion of this acid via the kidneys. The anti-inflammatory action helps to ease the pain caused by this condition and at the same time treats the cause by enhancing the elimination of the uric acid.

digestive system
Like many other seeds, for example Cardamom and Caraway, Celery seed is a gentle tonic to the digestion and the seeds can be sprinkled directly on to salads.

contraindications
None known.

preparations and dosage
tea 1 teaspoon per cup, infuse for 15 minutes and drink three times daily.

tincture 1 part herb to 5 parts 45% alcohol. Take 5ml in water three times daily. As this herb enhances the action of the kidneys eliminatory function it is wise to drink 2–3 litres of water a day while taking it.

combinations
Celery seed combines well with Meadowsweet, Devils claw, and Ginger to relieve symptoms of arthritis.

chamomile, german

Matricaria recutita

parts used
Flowers.

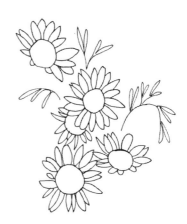

collection
The flowers should be collected between May and August when they are not wet with dew or rain. They need to be dried with care at not too high a temperature.

cultivation
This plant looks great planted in cracks between paving stones or

made into an ornamental lawn or even an aromatic bench seat. It is easy to find at garden centres, especially in early summer.

constituents
Volatile oil containing chamazulene. mucilage, coumarin, flavone glycosides,

actions
anti-inflammatory, anti-microbial (staphyloccous aureus), antiseptic (mild), anti-peptic ulcer, anodyne (mild), antispasmodic, bitter, carminative, vulnerary.

indications
nervous system
A relaxing herb which calms feelings of stress, anxiety, frustration, anger and tension: it is good for angry and teething children. It can also be used as a tea to drink before bed to aid sleep and prevent nightmares.

digestive system
Inflammations in the stomach and bowel are often made worse by stress and anxiety. Therefore chamomile is doubly useful in treating such complaints, as an antispasmodic, anti-inflammatory, calminative herb it is almost always a part of the successful treatment of indigestion, gastritis, inflammation, gingivitis, flatulence, dyspepsia and travel sickness.

respiratory system
As an anti-inflammatory the cold tea can be used as a wash for inflamed, sore eyes caused by hayfever or other irritants. It also acts as a mild antihistamine and used internally can be of benefit in the treatment of allergenic asthma and hayfever.

genitourinary system
Chamomile soothes premenstrual tension. As an antispasmodic the essential oil is beneficial when applied to the lower back and abdomen to alleviate painful spasms associated with periods. In a sitz bath the tea can reduce inflammation caused by thrush.

contraindications
None. Very rarely, however, Chamomile can cause allergy in the form of a skin rash when applied externally.

preparations and dosage
tea 1 teaspoon per cup, drink freely, or use cool as an eye wash.
tincture 1 part herb to 5 parts 45 % alcohol. Take 5ml in water three times daily.

sitz bath 25g in 2 litres of water, infuse for 20 minutes and add to sitz bath water. This is useful for soothing inflammation of the genitals, perineum and anus.

enema use 15g per 2 litres of water, infuse and cool to body temperature. A gentle bowel stimulant and soothing to the membrane of the lower intestine.

bath add 5 drops of essential oil to bath water to aid relaxation, relax menstrual spasm and ease backache.

cream add the essential oil or tincture to a base at 1–5% depending on requirement.

infused oil 15g dried herb to 300ml olive oil, leave in a glass jar in a sunny place for four days, strain and use for massage or add to a cream base.

combinations

For sore eyes it mixes well with Eyebright. For inflammation of the digestive system it mixes well with Peppermint, Marshmallow Root and Lemon balm. For hayfever it works well with Nettle, Eyebright, Elderflower and Peppermint. To aid sleep it mixes well with Lemon balm and Passion flower.

chickweed

Stellaria media

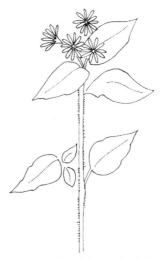

parts used
Fresh or dried aerial parts.

collection
Chickweed is a very common weed and can be collected all year round although it is most abundant in the spring and least in the winter.

cultivation
Chickweed is usually found as a weed and I can find no helpful instructions on its cultivation – it is prolific enough without help!

constituents
Saponin, glycosides, coumarins, flavonoids, vitamin C.

actions
Anti-rheumatic, vulnerary, emollient, antihistamine, alterative, mild laxative, refrigerant, cools excess body heat.

indications
skin

Chickweed is most commonly used externally as a remedy for hot, itchy skin complaints. It is the most powerful anti-itch remedy I have ever found. It works on any itch from eczema to mosquito bites. It can be applied as a cream, or made into an infusion and added to the bath water if larger areas of skin are affected.

musculoskeletal system

Chickweed has a reputation as an anti-rheumatic herb when used internally. It can also be applied to inflamed gouty joints as a poultice or ointment.

contraindications

None known.

preparations and dosage

tea 2 teaspoons of dried or fresh herb infused for 5 minutes, drink three cups daily.

bath use 25g of herb in 2 litres of water, infuse for 20 minutes and add to cool bath water to relieve hot, itchy skin.

tincture 1 part herb to 5 parts 45% alcohol. Take 2–3 ml in water, three times daily.

infused oil fill a jar or other container with Chickweed, press well down and cover with oil. Steep for two weeks, strain and bottle.

combinations

To make an extra emollient ointment, blend with Marshmallow root. As an anti-itch and anti-inflammatory cream for insect bites use blended with 1% Lavender essential oil. For internal use as an antirheumatic combine with Dandelion root and Celery seed.

chili

Capsicum spp.

parts used

Ripe or dried fruits.

collection

This is usually grown in tropical and subtropical countries so collection is usually from your local shops or the market.

cultivation

The plants are easily available from garden centres now and can be grown on a warm windowsill or in a greenhouse over the summer. Kew Gardens has a fantastic display of different varieties in the water lily house; from the classic Scotch Bonnet to some very beautiful purple and yellow varieties. Some varieties can grow up to 6ft high.

constituents

Capsaicin, oleic acid, palmitic acid, stearic acid, carotenoids, flavanoids, vitamin C.

actions

Circulatory stimulant, externally used as a rubefacient. It is also astringent, antiseptic and diuretic.

indications

circulatory system

Chili is especially useful for any condition where you need to strengthen and stimulate the function of the circulatory system, for example where you suffer from cold hands and feet or risk chilblains.

gastrointestinal system

A tonic for the digestion but can be too warming for some people so use with caution.

musculoskeletal system

Used externally as a rubefacient to relieve pain related to joint or muscle discomfort, for example for osteoarthritis or rheumatic pains.

contraindications

This herb can sometimes irritate and it most commonly effects the digestive system. It may irritate the lining of the stomach with its heating quality. Avoid in cases where a previous allergy to this herb is known or where there is inflammation in the gastrointestinal system.

preparations and dosage

tea use half to 1 teaspoon per cup, infuse for 10 minutes and use 1 tablespoon of this mixture in a cup of water. Drink as required.

tincture 1 part herb to 5 parts 45% alcohol, infuse for four days, macerate daily. Take a few drops in water three times daily.

combinations
Use in tiny doses to add to any tincture blend to help the herbs circulate through the whole body. It can be used in single doses to stimulate an individual mentally or energetically – try adding a little to your food and you will notice what a stimulating an effect it has, primarily on the circulation.

cleavers

Gallium aperine

parts used
Aerial parts.

collection
The aerial parts of the plant are collected before flowering and should be dried in a warm, shaded area.

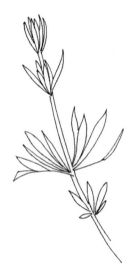

cultivation
Cleavers is a common weed and readily available in most gardens.

constituents
Glycoside asperuloside, gallotannic acid, citric acid, anthraquinone, flavonoids, iridoids, polyphonic acids.

actions
Lymphatic alterative and detoxifier, diuretic, astringent tonic, non-steroidal anti-inflammatory, adaptogen, anti-neoplastic

indications
lymphatic system
Cleavers is one of the most effective herbs for treating the lymphatic system. As an alterative it cleanses the lymphatic system and as a diuretic it helps to clear oedema. It can be used to reduce inflammation in swollen glands, for example, tonsillitis or glandular fever. It also has a reputation for making you thin and would certainly be a beneficial herb to use while dieting and to help clear cellulite.

urinary system
Cleavers is also helpful in cleansing the kidneys. It has a reputation as a stone solvent and has been used traditionally to treat kidney stones (gravel).

skin
It is a wonderfully cleansing herb and in this way is of great benefit for treating skin complaints from psoriasis to acne. It will cleanse the body and help to hydrate the skin.

contraindications
None known.

preparations and dosage
tea 2–3 teaspoons of the dried herb, or 4 teaspoons if it's fresh, infuse for 15 minutes and drink three cups daily.

fresh juice up to 3 teaspoonfuls three times daily. More can be used in severe cases.

tincture 1 part Cleavers to 5 parts 45% alcohol. Take 5ml in water three times daily.

combinations
For the lymphatic system combine with Red clover, Echinacea and Marigold. For cystitis or kidney stones (gravel) combine with a demulcent such as Marshmallow root and an anti-microbial such as Uva ursi. For acne and spots combine with Dandelion root and Marigold.

comfrey

Symphytum officinalis

parts used
Leaf and root.

collection
The leaves can be collected throughout the growing season, and the roots are unearthed during spring or autumn when the allantonin levels are at their highest. Split the roots down the middle and dry in a moderate oven with a temperature of 40–60°C for two to three hours.

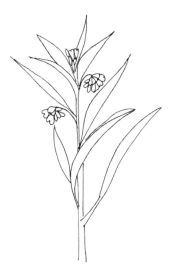

cultivation
Comfrey is easy to grow from root stock, which is usually bought as a green garden fertilizer. Once it is established it will be difficult to get rid of so feel free to chop back harshly when required.

constituents
Allantonin, Pyrrolizadine alkaloids, tannins, resin, essential oil, mucilage, phenolic acids, steroidal saponins (roots).

actions
Vulnerary, demulcent, astringent, expectorant, haemostatic,

indications
skin
Comfrey is a rapid healer of skin, bone and any other connective tissue, including the stomach and lungs as they have an interface with the external environment. It works so fast because it accelerates cell-division and is also demulcent and soothing. It can be used directly on the skin for any wound that needs this kind of healing and also internally for stomach ulcers, broken bones and tissue repair in recovery from operations.

respiratory system
It is useful in treating dry lung conditions as a soothing demulcent and expectorant, but it should not be used where there is oedema affecting the lungs.

contraindications
The root cannot now to be sold as an internal medicine due to the pyrrolizadine alkaloid content, which is thought to be toxic to the liver.

preparations and dosage
tea 1–3 teaspoons of the dry herb, infuse for 15 minutes and drink three times daily.

tincture 1 part herb to 5 parts 45% alcohol. Take 2–4ml in water three times daily. It is advised to take no more than 100ml in total per week and not to take for more than eight weeks at a time. If in any doubt consult a professional medical herbalist.

poultice the fresh root can be liquidised, or bashed with a rolling pin, to make a poultice which can be applied externally to any area requiring an increase in tissue regeneration.

infused oil use fresh leaf or root and cover with a good quality oil, extra virgin olive is ideal, infuse in sunlight for eight days, strain and apply as a massage oil when required.

ointment 1 part powder to 10 parts ointment base of your choice, apply as required.

combinations
For a powerful anti-infective skin healing ointment blend with Myrrh powder. As a tea for a dry cough use with Echinacea and Sage.

coriander

Coriandrum sativum

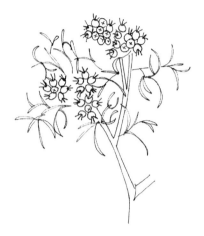

parts used
Seed, flowering tops and leaves.

collection
Collect in late summer and allow the seed to ripen before collection, if necessary.

cultivation
An annual herb growing to a height of one metre with delicate, bright green leaves and umbels of white flowers which progress to form light brown, round seed heads. Prefers germinating on a hot bed in rich soil. Slugs seem to love this herb so protect it well.

constituents
The essential oil contains: alcohols including linalol and thymol,. esters including linalyl actate, terpenes including caryophyllene, α-pinene, limonene & β-phellandrene and many other trace compounds.

actions
Analgesic, antibacterial, antidepressive, anti-infectious, antirheumatic, antispasmodic, aperitive, aphrodisiac, carminative, circulatory tonic, digestive stimulant, neurotonic, stomachic, general tonic.

indications
musculoskeletal system
The essential oil can be used to relieve muscle spasm and, acting as an antirheumatic, help to relieve the symptoms of rheumatism and arthritis.

circulatory system
A gentle tonic for treating poor circulation.

digestive system
This herb can help to balance the digestive function by calming spasm and encouraging healthy digestion. It is useful for constipation or diarrhoea and abdominal or epigastric distention.

nervous system
As a general tonic it helps to support mental function, particularly concentration and memory. On a psychological level this is a spicy, aphrodisiac tonic used to reawaken a passion for life, yet it is also grounding and comforting.

contraindications
Non-toxic, safe in prescribed doses.

preparations and dosage
essential oil use up to 5 drops in a bath or use in a burner to change the atmosphere. It can also be added in a low dose (up to 1%) to a blend of oils for massage treatments.

tea use 1 teaspoon dried seed per cup, infuse for 10 minutes and drink up to three times daily.

tincture 1 part herb/seed to 5 parts 45% alcohol, infuse for two weeks, macerate daily. Take 2ml in water three times daily.

combinations
Use in an essential oil blend to help tonify a tired and worried person. Blend with jasmine and orange essential oils, use as a massage, in a burner to scent the room or in a bath to uplift, relax and nourish the spirit. Use to flavour foods, from salads or paella to curries, as a general nerve and digestive tonic.

cornsilk

Zea mays

parts used
The stigmas from the female flowers of maize, which are the fine, soft threads, about 10–20cm long.

collection
The stigmas can be collected from the ripened fruit: corn on the cob. The Cornsilk is the soft thready part which you normally throw away when preparing the cob for consumption.

cultivation

Corn likes a very sunny position and rich, slightly acidic soil. Sow seeds outside 2–3cm deep, 5–6cm apart once soil temperatures are consistently above 10°C. Plant in clusters rather than rows for best results and repeat the sowing every two weeks for a continuous crop throughout the season. When they are 6–7cm tall, thin the plants out to about 30cm apart. Mulch them when the ground has warmed up to help them stay moist and weed free.

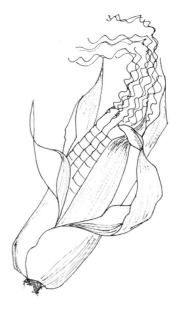

constituents

Saponins, vitamin C and K, a volatile alkaloid, sterols, allantonin, tannin.

actions

Diuretic, demulcent, tonic, soothing to the urinary system, antilithic.

indications
urinary system

Cornsilk is useful as a soothing demulcent for any form of irritation to the urinary system including: cystitis, lack of control in bladder function, bed wetting, irritation of the urinary tract due to uric and phosphatic acids, urethritis, and to aid expulsion of kidney stones (gravel). It can also be used as temporary relief for the pain associated with nephritis.

contraindications

None.

preparations and dosage

tea herbalists believe infusing corn silk is the best way to use this herb. Use 2–3 teaspoons per cup, infuse for 15 minutes and drink freely. I have used capsules successfully for children who refuse to drink herb teas although it could also easily be mixed with fruit juice to disguise the flavour and encourage consumption.

combinations

It works especially well with Marshmallow leaf for treating inflammation and irritation of the bladder. If there is infection then it is best mixed with antimicrobial herbs such as Echinacea, Thyme or Golden rod.

dandelion

Taraxacum officinalis

parts used
Leaves, root.

collection
The roots are best collected between June and August when they are at their bitterest. Split them longitudinally before drying. The leaves may be collected at any time.

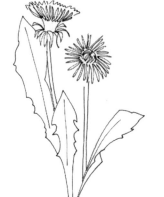

constituents
Glycosides, terpenoids, choline, up to 5% potassium, carotenoids, sesquiterpene lactones, vitamins A, B and C.

cultivation
I have never needed to cultivate this plant as there are always so many in the lawn for me to extract! Let the lawn grow to a reasonable length and their flowers will highlight their position so you can harvest them easily over the summer period.

actions
leaf powerful diuretic, urinary antiseptic.
root bitter tonic, pancreatic regulator, galactagogue, antirheumatic, pancreatic and bile duct stimulant, stimulant to the portal circulation, mild laxative. Promotes elimination of plasma cholesterol.

indications
urinary system
The leaf is of most benefit here as it is slightly more diuretic than the root and is a urinary antiseptic, although the root also has some diuretic properties. Its action is comparable to the drug 'Frusemide'. Drugs which stimulate diuresis also cause a loss of potassium, which will, unfortunately, aggravate any heart problem for which the diuretic is used. Dandelion leaf, however, contains such appreciable amounts of potassium it compensates for the loss and is therefore a very balanced remedy for treating oedema caused by heart problems.

digestive system

The root is used as a cholagogue for inflammation and congestion of the liver and gall-bladder and to counter any tendency toward gall stones. It also helps to improve pancreatic function and reduce any tendency towards hypoglycaemia (the need to eat every few hours to maintain energy levels). Its ability to promote bile flow also gives the root its action as a mild laxative.

musculoskeletal system

Its action on the digestive system, of improving digestion and elimination, makes it beneficial for arthritic and rheumatic conditions which often stem from poor digestive function.

contraindications

It should not be used where the bile duct is blocked.

preparations and dosage

tea leaf, use 2 teaspoons fresh or dried per cup, brew for 15 minutes and drink three times daily. The fresh leaves can also be eaten raw as a salad vegetable.

decoction 2 teaspoons per cup, boil the root for 20 minutes and drink three times daily.

tincture 1 part of the root and leaf to 5 parts 45% alcohol. Take 5ml tincture in water three times daily.

dandelion coffee drink freely.

combinations

Use as a treatment for cystitis by combining with a demulcent herb such as Marshmallow leaf and an immune stimulant herb such as Elderflower, Echinacea or Calendula. To improve liver function use the root in equal parts with Milk thistle.

echinacea

Echinacea purpurea, Echinacea angustifolia

parts used

Purpurea – whole plant, angustifolia – roots.

collection

The roots should be unearthed in the autumn, the tops can be harvested when flowering.

cultivation

A beautiful addition to any garden scheme the tall, purple-flowered daisy-like bloom is easy to grow from seed or root stock. Sow in either autumn or spring in the open ground. Prefers a sunny position.

constituents
In angustifolia – Echinacosides, also alkaloids, polysaccharides, flavonoids, essential oil.

actions
Immune stimulant, antimicrobial, alterative, blood cleanser, lymphatic, raises white blood cell count, stimulates killer cells that resist foreign bacteria, vulnerary

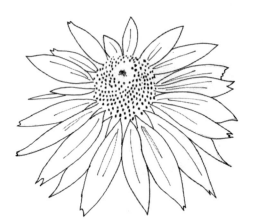

indications
immune system
Echinacea is well known for its ability to boost the immune system and is one of the most popular remedies for this purpose. It is effective against both viral and bacterial attacks affecting any part of the body, for example: cystitis, gastritis, food poisoning, otitis, septicaemia, boils, gingivitis, colds, flus. It can also be used to help support a compromised immune system deal with the effects of vaccination. Echinacea angustifolia was traditionally called 'snake bite' by the native Mohawk and Cherokee American Indians as they used it to detoxify the poison in the bloodstream following snake bites.

contraindications
None known.

preparations and dosage
tea use 1 teaspoon of the root or tops, simmer for 15 minutes and drink three times daily.
tincture 1part herb to 5 parts 45% alcohol. Take 2–4ml in water three times daily.

combinations
For the treatment of cystitis use combined with Marshmallow leaf or Cornsilk, Yarrow and Uva ursi. For flu and colds it works well with Thyme, Yarrow, Elderflower and Sage. As a treatment for acne, to cleanse the blood and lymphatic system, mix it with Blue flag iris root and Calendula.

elder

Sambucus nigra

parts used
Flowers and berries.

collection
The flowers can be collected in spring and early summer and dried as rapidly as possible in the shade. The berries are collected in August and September.

cultivation
This is a small tree, which some consider a weed, so you may not wish to introduce it into the garden. It is always to be found in hedgerows and parks. There are, however, many beautiful, ornamental varieties with either golden or purple foliage which will brighten any colour scheme.

constituents
Flowers contain flavonoids including rutin, tannins, essential oil. Berries also contain vitamin C and iron.

actions
anti-inflammatory, laxative (especially berries) anticatarrhal, diaophoretic, diuretic, urinary antiseptic.

indications
respiratory system
A blocked nose and painful sinuses respond well to Elder flower and berry. The berry is thought to be more warming and therefore

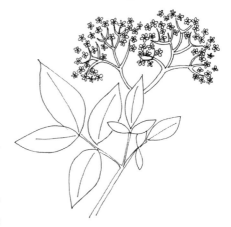

more appropriate for winter colds and flu while the flower is more appropriate for hayfever congestion and summer colds and flu. It is also diaphoretic and can be useful in reducing fevers, especially for children with viral infections of the upper respiratory tract. 5ml of the tincture or syrup can be taken daily throughout the winter season as a prophylactic treatment, to prevent colds and flu in winter,

urinary system
As a diuretic and mild urinary antiseptic, Elderflower can be combined with other demulcent and anti-infective herbs to ease cystitis.

contraindications
None known.

preparations and dosage
tea 2 teaspoons of the flowers or berries, infuse for 15 minutes. For acute conditions drink every 2 hours, otherwise three times daily.

tincture 1 part herb to 5 parts 45% alcohol, Take 2–4 ml in water three times daily, again in acute situations this dose can be taken every two hours.

combinations
For hayfever it blends well with Eyebright, Nettle and Chamomile. For sinusitis mix it with Plantain and Peppermint. For winter flu blend the Elderberry with Thyme, Echinacea and Marshmallow leaf..

eyebright
Euphrasia Officinalis

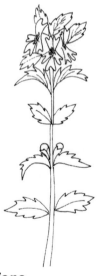

parts used
Dried aerial parts.

collection
Collect the aerial parts of the plant while in bloom in late summer to autumn. It should be dried in an airy place.

cultivation
Tolerates a wide range of soil and conditions but prefers to grow in grassland rather than in a garden setting.

constituents
Tannin, iridoid glycosides, essential oil, resins.

actions
Anti-inflammatory, anti-catarrhal, astringent, anti-histamine.

indications
respiratory system

Eyebright is an excellent herb for treating the respiratory system. It can treat sinusitis and allergic inflammatory responses due to its anti-histamine and anti-inflammatory actions and will alleviate sore eyes, itchy throat and other hayfever-type symptoms. As an anti-catarrhal it can help to relieve the runny nose caused by allergy or viral infection, especially where there is post-nasal drip causing a cough and phlegm in the throat. The herb can be used internally or, for inflamed sore eyes, the tea can be cooled and used as a very soothing eye wash.

contraindications

None known.

preparations and dosage

tea 1 teaspoon per cup, brew for 10 minutes and drink freely. If using the tea as an eye wash do ensure that it is strained well, so no 'bits' can get in the eye, and that it is cooled thoroughly.

tincture 1 part herb to 5 parts 45% alcohol. Take 2–6ml in water three times daily.

combinations

To relieve hayfever and allergy affecting the respiratory system, blend with Nettle, Chamomile and Peppermint. For sinusitis add it to a mix of Elderflower and Plantain. It can also be mixed with Chamomile tea and used as an eye wash.

fennel

Foeniculum vulgare

parts used

Seed, leaves.

collection

The seed should be harvested in autumn when it is ripe. The brown umbel can be cut off and the seeds removed. The seeds should be dried in a warm, shady place. The leaves can be collected fresh for use as a tea or dried and collected any time throughout the growing season.

cultivation

It is easy to grow, prefers full sun and is very hardy and easily grown from seed. Sow the seeds into the herb or vegetable

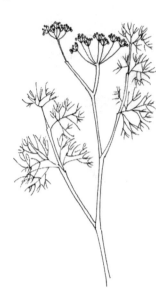

garden early in the season and cover them with 1cm of soil. Thin the plants to 25–30cm apart, in rows 35–40cm apart once they are large enough to handle. Re-sow again in summer for a second harvest in autumn.

constituents

6% essential oil, containing fenchone, anethole. Fatty oil at 10%, coumarins, sterols and flavonoids

actions

A gentle warming agent for delicate stomachs, carminative, anti-spasmodic, galactagogue, digestive tonic, orexigenic (stimulates appetite), mild stimulant, antimicrobial, anticoagulant (vitamin K antagonist), expectorant, phyto-oestrogen activity, rubefacient.

indications

digestive system

Fennel's main use is in treating the digestive system. It works to disperse excess wind and is especially useful for colic in infants. It can be drunk as a tea by the mother and the properties of the fennel are passed through the breast milk directly to the child, aiding digestion and reducing the tendency to produce wind and colic symptoms. Interestingly, it also helps increase the flow of breast milk in nursing mothers. It can also stimulate the appetite and soothe and relax irritable bowels.

musculoskeletal system

Fennel can be used externally as a rub for inflamed joints. Its warming, rubefacient activity increases circulation to the area, helping to remove toxins via the blood and relieve deeper inflammation.

contraindications

As it has phyto-oestrogenic properties some sources consider it should be avoided if there has been a history of breast cancer. It is also contraindicated during pregnancy due to its hormonal action.

preparations and dosage
tea fresh or dried leaves, 1 teaspoon per cup, brew for 10 minutes and drink three times daily. For infants, give just 2–3 teaspoons of the tea at this strength.

aromatic water 5–15 drops, before food, to aid digestion.

tincture 1 part Fennel seed to 5 parts 45% alcohol, Take 2–4ml in water three times daily.

essential oil to make a gentle massage oil for stomach cramps use 2–3 drops in 5ml oil. To use as a rubefacient on a small area use 10 drops in 5ml oil.

combinations
For poor digestion and flatulence it blends well with Chamomile. To improve the flow of breast milk it can be mixed with Milk thistle.

ginger
Zingiber officinalis

parts used
Root stock or rhizome.

collection
The root stock is dug up once the leaves have dried. The remains of the stem and root fibre are removed and then it is dried in the sun. As ginger doesn't grow in this country, unless you have a very hot greenhouse, it is probably best collected from the shops or market.

cultivation
I have grown this herb simply by planting a shop bought rhizome and burying it a few centimetres deep in rich, houseplant compost then leaving in a warm windowsill in full sun to mimic its natural conditions as best I can.

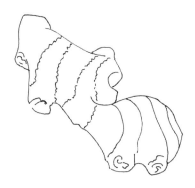

constituents
Essential oil, gingerols, phenolic compounds, mucilage.

actions
Anti-inflammatory, carminative, antispasmodic, expectorant, vasodilator, anti-cholesterol, circulatory stimulant, antiemetic, diaphoretic.

indications
digestive system
Ginger is one of the best remedies for all kinds of nausea, vomiting, travel sickness, morning sickness, viral gastroenteritis and food poisoning. The powder, taken in capsules, works best for this purpose although sipping ginger tea made from the rhizome brings immediate relief. As an antispasmodic it is helpful for relieving the stomach cramps associated with retching. It also acts as a carminative, aiding digestion and helping to reduce wind production in the bowel.

circulatory system
Ginger is a warming herb and is a perfect remedy for people who suffer from poor circulation and who feel the cold. It is also thought to be an aphrodisiac, perhaps partly because it improves circulation throughout the body, but also because it restores our fire and passion for life.

musculoskeletal system
The essential oil is a wonderful treatment for aching muscles and joints, especially after gardening in cold weather. Add a few drops to bath water or add to a base oil or cream and apply to the affected areas.

contraindications
None known.

preparations and dosage
capsules 2 capsules every hour in acute cases of sickness. When you use ginger capsules you cannot taste them as you swallow them but it is interesting to note that you can sometimes taste it in your mouth some time after ingesting the capsule. This is because the aromatic components in the ginger has been circulated by the blood system and reached your mouth and taste buds that way, giving a sensation similar to the taste of ginger. It is said that when you can taste this 'flavour' of ginger after swallowing a few ginger capsules then you know that you have had a dose which should be medicinally effective.

tea chop up about 1cm of rhizome and pour boiling water over the top. The rhizome sinks to the bottom of the cup so there is no need to strain it like other herb teas.

tincture Take 30 drops in water three times daily.

combinations

As an external treatment for muscular aches use the essential oil of Ginger with Juniper Berry: use about 30 drops in 30ml of oil for local topical applications. As a delicious warming and immune stimulating, digestive tonic tea, use the rhizome with lemon juice and add honey if there is also a sore throat. Ginger can be used in conjunction with any herb where you need to make sure the herbs get to the right part of the body as it stimulates the circulation and therefore the distribution of the other herbs taken will be enhanced.

hawthorn

Crataegus monogyna

parts used
Flowers and berries.

collection
The flowers are collected in May and the berries in September and October.

cultivation
Hawthorn can be used as a hedging plant or a small, ornamental tree. It comes in several varieties with pink, red and white-flowered varieties. It is very easy to grow and easy to find at garden centres.

constituents
Saponins, glycosides, flavonoids, ascorbic acid, tannin

actions
Cardiac tonic, blood pressure normaliser, antispasmodic, sedative to nervous system.

indications
circulatory system

Hawthorn is the top herb for treating any condition affecting the circulatory system. It has a tonic effect on the heart, improving blood flow to and through the heart. It strengthens the heart muscle, without increasing the beats per minute or raising blood pressure, and it enhances stamina. It works to normalise blood pressure whether raised or reduced. It is also a mild sedative, mainly for use when anxiety causes heart palpitations, and can be used as a preventive.

contraindications

This herb has the potential to increase the action of heart medication so, if prescribed medicine is being taken, always consult a medical herbalist for safety advice before using it.

preparations and dosage

tea leaves and flowers, use 2 teaspoons per cup, infuse for 10 minutes and drink three times daily.

decoction fruits, use 2 teaspoons per cup, simmer gently for 5 minutes and drink three times daily.

tincture 1 part herb to 5 parts 45% alcohol. Take 2–4ml in water three times daily.

combinations

To treat anxiety affecting the heart use with Rose and Lemon balm. For poor circulation use with Rosemary.

horse chestnut

Aesculus hippocastrum

parts used

'Conkers', the chestnut, the brown seed.

collection

The ripe chestnuts should be collected as they fall from the trees in September and October.

cultivation

This is huge tree when it reaches maturity. It has beautiful pink or white flowers in late spring and is well worth a place in a garden which has the space to accommodate it.

constituents

Flavones, Saponin, tannin, starch, fatty oil, glycosides; aesculin.

actions
Astringent, circulatory tonic, anti-inflammatory, vasodilator, tones and protects blood vessels, anti-oedema. Stimulates production of prostaglandin F-alpha which contracts veins.

indications
circulatory system
The action of Horse chestnut is quite unique; it seems to strengthen and tone the veins by increasing their integrity and ability to hold blood. It can be used internally and externally to treat varicose veins, piles and oedema caused by trauma or weakness of the venous system.

contraindications
Although this herb is used as fodder for animals it is not really edible and should always be used with care as a medicine since excess or inappropriate use could cause mild poisoning and stomach cramps. Safe doses and preparations are listed below.

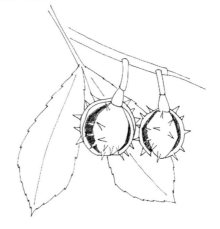

preparations and dosage
average dose 1–2g daily

tea half a teaspoon of dried Horse chestnut powder per cup, infuse for 15 minutes, use half to 1 cup three times daily. This tea can also be used, once it has cooled, as a wash for external use on haemorrhoids or varicose veins.

tincture 1 part powder, or finely chopped Horse chestnut to 10 parts 45% tincture. Macerate for 8 days before filtering. Take 5ml in water daily.

cream a cream or ointment can be prepared for use on varicose veins and haemorrhoids by adding the tincture.

combinations
For varicose veins and piles it combines well with hawthorn and yarrow as a tincture taken internally. For external treatment of piles and varicose veins it can be used with Witch hazel and Marigold.

hyssop

Hysopus officinalis

parts used
Dried aerial parts.

collection
Collect the flowering tops in August.

cultivation
This is an evergreen herb growing 1–2 feet tall. Naturalised to Britain it grows very successfully in soil with good drainage and a sunny position.

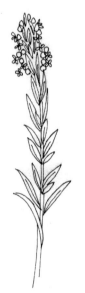

constituents
1% volatile oil, flavanoid, glycosides, diosmin, tannin. Essential oil also consists of ketones including isopinocamphone and pinocamphone. Terpenes including β-pinene, β-caryophyllene and germacrene. Methyl-ether phenols including myrtenyl methyl ether and methyl chavicol. Alcohols including nerolidol plus many other trace compounds.

actions
Antibacterial, anticatarrhal, anti-infectious, antirheumatic, antiseptic, antiviral, decongestant, diuretic, expectorant, immune tonic, mucolytic, neurotonic, general tonic.

indications
respiratory system
The primary use of Hyssop is for treating problems associated with infection of the respiratory system: especially where it relates to infection of the lungs. It has an immune tonic effect and in addition works directly on infections as an antibacterial and antiviral. Its expectorant and mucolytic action will encourage elimination of phlegm and clearing of the chest.

nervous system
This is a stimulating neurotonic, which helps to relieve mental and physical lethargy and alleviate depression and moodiness. It

stimulates the mind, helping us to be fully awake, engaged and able to face the world.

contraindications

The essential oil has a high percentage of potentially neurotoxic ketones and should not be used by pregnant or breastfeeding mothers, children under the age of two, epileptics or if suffering from fever. It should be used with maximum dosage diluted to 2%.

preparations and dosage

tea use 1–2 teaspoons per cup, infuse for 10 minutes and drink three times daily.

tincture 1 part herb to 5 parts 45% alcohol, infuse for 2 weeks, macerate daily. Take 3ml in water three times daily.

combinations

It can be used to treat coughs and bronchitis with demulcent herbs such as Marshmallow leaf and a further immune tonic such as Echinacea or Elderflower. In treatment of the nervous system use as a tonic with Lemon balm and Borage.

juniper

Juniperus communis

parts used
Dried ripe berry.

collection
The ripe, unshrivelled berries are collected in the autumn and dried slowly in the shade, to avoid loosing the essential oil component.

cultivation
This small tree is either male or female and both are needed to produce the juniper berries prized in herbal medicine. A beautiful, blue, ornamental conifer.

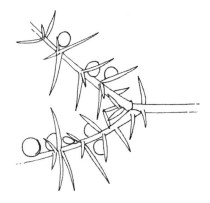

constituents
Essential oil, monoterpenes, sesquiterpenes, invert sugar, flavone, glycosides, resin, tannin, vitamin C.

actions
Urinary antiseptic, stimulating diuretic, digestive tonic, emmenagogue, parasiticide (externally), carminative, antirheumatic.

indications
musculoskeletal system
Juniper's bitter action increases digestion and aids elimination whilst also working on elimination via the kidneys. It therefore helps to detoxify the body of the toxins that cause the inflammatory pain of arthritis.

urinary system
This is a useful urinary antiseptic for cases of cystitis. The essential oil can also be rubbed over the kidney area in the small of the back to tonify kidney function and act as a general tonic.

contraindications
It is contraindicated in pregnancy and kidney disease.

preparations and dosage
tea 1 teaspoon of crushed berries per cup, infuse for 30 minutes, drink three times daily.

tincture 1 part herb to 5 parts 45% alcohol. Take 1–2ml in water three times daily.

essential oil 10 drops in 5ml of base oil as a local rub for the kidneys or on arthritic joints.

40 berry detox This traditional French detox starts with eating just one berry on the first day, two berries on the the second, three on the third and so on until the fortieth day when you eat forty berries. The process is then reversed until you are back to zero again.

combinations
As an essential oil combination for arthritis it blends especially well with Ginger. As a urinary antiseptic it should be blended with a demulcent such as Marshmallow or Cornsilk.

lavender

Lavandula angustifolia

parts used
Flowers.

collection
The flowers should be collected just before they open between June and September. They need to be dried gently at a

temperature below 35°C to prevent loss of the essential oil component.

cultivation
Lavender likes full sun, good drainage, rich soil and not too much water; overwatering reduces the aromatic properties. In fact the rougher you treat this plant the better it is supposed to smell! It is easy to grow from cuttings but not so easy to grow from seed.

constituents
Essential oil, linalol, geraniol, cineole, limonene, sesquiterpenes, flavonoids, coumarins, triterpenes

actions
antidepressive, antispasmodic, antiseptic, carminative, sedative, anticonvulsant, antimicrobial,

indications
nervous system
Lavender's primary actions are on the nervous system as an antidepressive, calming, antispasmodic herb. The essential oil is very powerful and used in a bath at night can be of great benefit to encourage a good night's sleep. The oil can also be applied directly to the temples to relieve a headache or migraine. As an antispasmodic the oil can be blended with a base oil and massaged into the affected area, whether this is a muscle, the abdomen or lower back. The herb itself is a little bitter and floral tasting but there are recipes for Lavender shortbread (see Page 144) and scones which make a very pleasant remedy for depression. The herb can be drunk as a tea, or the tincture and aromatic water can be used internally.

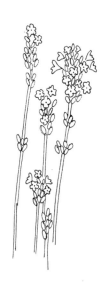

skin
Its cooling and vulnerary action help to heal scars and especially burns, once they have been cooled under water of course. It also has antiseptic properties and the essential oil can be used diluted on cuts and grazes.

contraindications

Very rarely skin allergy may occur. If this happens discontinue use immediately.

preparations and dosage

tea 1 teaspoon per cup and drink three times daily.

tincture 1 part herb to 5 parts 45% alcohol. Take 5ml in water three times daily.

bath add 5–10 drops of the essential oil to the bath water, mix well.

massage oil add 10 drops per 15ml of oil.

combinations

To blend a relaxing bath oil use Lavender with Geranium. To soothe aching muscles, especially for gardeners, use Rosemary. As a treatment for depression blend it with Borage, Lemon balm and Peppermint.

lemon

Citrus limonum

parts used

Fruit and epicarp.

collection

It is probably easiest to collect the fruit from the shops, unless you have a sunny conservatory where you can store the plant over winter.

cultivation

All citrus trees are happy in the summer in Britain and quite enjoy the changes in temperature: it causes them to flower and consequently fruit more often. But they do need to be protected from the frosts over winter so you either need have space, ideally a sunny conservatory, to bring your favourite specimens inside or ensure they are well wrapped up for the winter period.

constituents

Lemon essential oil: terpenes, limonene, aldehydes, alcohols, coumarins and furocoumarins. Lemon juice: vitamin C, citric acid, sugar.

actions

Antibacterial, aerial antiseptic, antifungal, antirheumatic, antispasmodic, carminative, digestive stimulant, immune tonic, lymphatic decongestant.

indications
digestive system
Lemon is a powerful carminative and the tea can be very effective for relieving nausea. The essential oil can be blended into an anti-microbial mouthwash to treat halitosis and gingivitis. It is also a powerful antispasmodic for the gut and is a traditional remedy for obstinate hiccups.

lymphatic system
Lemon and honey tea is a traditional remedy for sore throats. This is because it is a powerful lymphatic decongestant, has a high vitamin C content, helps to boost the immune system and is anti-microbial so that it kills off the bugs which cause sore throats.

skin
Lemon essential oil is active against the virus which causes veruccas, warts. The oil can be applied neat directly on to the affected area and a plaster laid over the top to prevent the oil being washed or rubbed off.

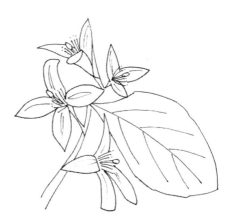

contraindications
The essential oil is phototoxic which means it should not be used on the skin if you are planning on being in the sun within twelve hours of its application. It is otherwise very safe. The essential oil should not be used internally.

preparations and dosage
tea infuse the fruit in slices, including the rind, or just use the juice and add hot water depending on your own taste. It is especially good with honey in the treatment of sore, inflamed throats.
essential oil used in 1% dilution, added to a base cream or oil for massage, this is especially good for lymphatic decongestion (and cellulite).

combinations
For a sore throat, blend the juice of half a lemon with a little chopped ginger and a teaspoon of honey in a cup of hot water. Infuse for 5–10 minutes and drink freely.

lemon balm

Melissa officinalis

parts used
Aerial parts, leaves and flowers.

collection
The leaves may be harvested two or three times a year between June and September. They are gathered by cutting off the young shoots when they are approximately 30cm long. They should be dried in the shade at a temperature not above 35°C.

cultivation
Extremely easy to grow from seed, lemon balm prefers full sun and a well drained but rich soil. It can be a little invasive once it gets comfortable so cut back ruthlessly to keep it under control.

constituents
Rich in essential oil containing citral, citronellal, geraniol, linalol, bitter principles, flavones, resins.

actions
Carminative, antispasmodic, antidepressive, hypotensive, diaphoretic, antihistamine, antiviral (the tea or aromatic water applied topically and particularly useful to treat herpes sores), nerve relaxant, anxiolytic.

indications
nervous system
As an anxiolytic, antidepressive, calminative herb it is one of the most useful for treating complaints affecting the nervous system. It can be used to relieve anxiety, depression, melancholy, nervous excitability, especially affecting the stomach or heart, panic attacks, palpitations and insomnia. It also calms anger, irritability and frustration, and helps to relieve feelings of loss and grief.

digestive system
Lemon balm's antispasmodic properties are beneficial for treating stomach cramps. As a carminative it is used to gently increase peristalsis and relieve bloating caused by wind.

circulatory system

As a calming herb, and also a hypotensive, it works to reduce raised blood pressure especially where it is made worse by stress and anger.

skin

Lemon balm has an antiviral action which is present in the water extract of the herb, i.e. in tea or aromatic water. It is specifically active against the herpes virus erupting as cold sores, shingles, chicken pox, genital warts and fever blisters. It also has an anti-bacterial action.

contraindications

None known.

preparations and dosage

tea 2 teaspoons of fresh or dried leaves per cup, drink freely.

tincture 1 part herb to 5 parts 45% alcohol. Take 2–6ml in water three times daily.

bath use 25g to 2 litres of water, infuse for 15 minutes and add to the bath water to aid sleep, calm anger, heal grief and reduce skin reaction to shingles and chicken pox.

aromatic water this is useful to treat Herpes simplex 1+2, oral and genital warts, and can also be useful as a general antiviral in chicken pox and shingles.

combinations

For stress and tension it combines well with Lime flower and Passionflower. For digestive complaints it combines well with Chamomile.

carmelite tea this is popular in France as an 'elixir of life', digestive and tonic for anaemia, poor appetite and low spirits.

3 litres spirits or wine,

500g fresh lemon balm leaves and flowers,

16g Angelica root,

125g Lemon peel,

200g Coriander,

40g Nutmeg,

4g cinnamon,

2g of Cloves.

Steep finely rubbed herbs and roots and powered seeds in spirits or wine for eight days in a dark place, stirring daily; decant, filter and bottle.

lime flower

Tilia spp.

parts used
Dried flowers.

collection
The flowers can be collected immediately after flowering in mid-summer. They should be collected on a dry day and dried carefully in the shade.

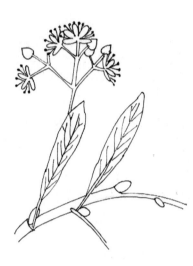

constituents
Essential oil, farnesol, mucilage, flavonoids, hesperidin, coumarin fraxoside, vanillin, tannins, phenolic acids.

cultivation
This is a very large tree at maturity and very common in Britain. You will probably remember parking your car under one as they drop a sticky substance in spring. If you have a large garden with enough space it is a very nice tree to have, otherwise you will no doubt find a specimen in your local park.

actions
Nervine, anti-spasmodic, diaphoretic, diuretic, mild astringent, hypotensive, sedative, anticoagulant, anxiolytic, immune enhancer indications

indications
nervous system
Lime flower is a mild relaxant, which is not as strong as Valerian and therefore more appropriate for children's sleep difficulties and nervous problems. It is specific for treating nervous palpitations sometimes associated with panic attacks.

cardiovascular system
This is a gentle hypotensive and prophylactic which can prevent development of arteriosclerosis and hypertension. Its relaxant effect on the cardiovascular system gives Lime flower a role in treating some forms of migraine.

immune system

As an immune enhancer and diaphoretic it is very useful in treating colds and flu especially when there is fever. It is gentle and effective for children and can be used to prevent febrile convulsions.

contraindications

None. However, if you do wish to treat high blood pressure with this herb please consult a medical herbalist first, especially if you are on medication. They will be able to monitor your progress and ensure the herb is right for you.

preparations and dosage

tea 1–2 teaspoons per cup, infuse for 10 minutes and drink three times daily.

tincture 1 part Lime flower to 5 parts 25% alcohol (white wine)., Macerate for 8 days. Take 5ml in water three times daily.

combinations

For nervous tension Lime flower combines beautifully with Lemon Balm. To treat raised blood pressure (if not on medication) it can be used with Hawthorn and Yarrow. To reduce fever combine with Elderflower and Echinacea.

marigold

Calendula officinalis

parts used

Flowers, leaves.

collection

Either the whole flower or just the petals are collected between June and September. The flowers and petals need to be dried quickly in a good current of warm air, spread out on sheets of paper, loosely without touching each other, or they lose their colour. Historically the leaves were also used and should only be picked when dry. The leaves are no longer used by herbalists but they are edible and can be used as salad leaves. The flowers can also be macerated in oil.

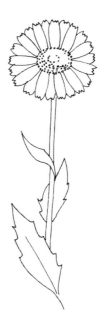

cultivation

It is very easy to grow from seed and prefers full sun but is tolerant of semi-shade. Sow in open ground in spring. This plant will self-seed from then on and the crop will expand very quickly so be prepared to cut it back hard when necessary.

constituents

Saponins, carotenoids, bitter principle, essential oil, sterols, flavonoids, mucilage, triterpenes.

actions

Anti-inflammatory, astringent, vulnerary, antifungal, cholagogue, emmenagogue, immune stimulant, anti-protazoal, antispasmodic, antihaemorrhage, antihistamine, antibacterial (particularly against staphylococcus and streptococcus), anthelmintic anti-emetic, anti-cancer, antiseptic, styptic, haemostatic, diaphoretic, , oestrogenic activity (extract from fresh flowers), menstrual regulator.

indications

respiratory system

As an anti-inflammatory, antibacterial immune stimulant Marigold is very effective as a gargle in treating enlarged and inflamed lymphatic glands.

digestive system

Its vulnerary action to the mucous membranes is very powerful and can be used internally to treat gastric and duodenal ulcers. As a cholagogue and choleretic it is effective in relieving symptoms of jaundice and gall bladder inflammation.

genitourinary system

Marigold is an emmenagogue and antispasmodic, perfect for regulating and tonifying the reproductive organs, and can be used to treat absent or painful periods. It can also be used internally and externally, as an immune stimulant and antifungal, to treat vaginal thrush.

skin

It is a great wound healer as it speeds up skin regeneration especially when using the 90% tincture. It is very effective for treating sores, ulcers, sore nipples in nursing mothers, varicose veins, chilblains, bee and wasp stings, fungal infections, thrush.

contraindications

None known.

preparations and dosage

tea 1–2 teaspoons of flowers per cup, infuse for 15 minutes and drink freely.

tincture 50g petals to 500ml 45% alcohol, stand for 14 days in a warm place, shake daily. Take 5–20 drops in water daily.

sitz bath to treat genital thrush use 25g to 2 litres of water, infuse for 20 minutes, add to bath water or a sitz bath and rest in the water for 10 minutes.

infused oil infuse flowers in a good quality oil for 2 weeks, strain and use as a massage oil or add to an ointment base.

cream add either the tincture or infused oil to a base cream.

ointment use 450g butter to 1.5 litres of marigold juice (extract this from the leaves using a juicer or with a pestle and mortar then squeeze the juice through a muslin to strain). Blend the butter and juice thoroughly and store in a glass jar in a cool place and use as required. This preparation will not store for as long as some other combinations but it is worth a try.

combinations

As a treatment for thrush, add the dried or fresh flowers to a sitz bath along with Lavender, Rose, Comfrey and Chamomile. To treat a sore throat use the diluted tincture mixed with Myrrh, Sage and Echinacea to gargle.

marshmallow

Althea officinalis

parts used
Leaves, root, flowers.

collection
The flowers are collected in summer, usually August. The leaves are picked in late summer after flowering. The root is collected in late autumn, cleaned of cork and root fibres and dried immediately.

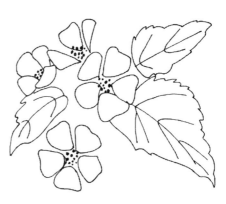

cultivation
A very robust perennial, tolerant of most sites and soils, which is easy to grow from seed. Sow the seed in open ground in spring.

constituents
Root 25–35% mucilage; pectin; tannin; asparagine.

actions
Root: demulcent, diuretic, emollient, vulnerary.
Leaf: demulcent, expectorant, diuretic, emollient.

indications
skin
The leaf and root can be powdered to make a useful drawing and healing poultice for application to boils and spots. It draws toxins out of the skin and helps to soothe inflammation and redness at the same time.

digestive system
The root is specific for treating inflammation of the digestive system including conditions such as gastritis and irritable bowel syndrome. It is very soothing so any irritation from food or allergy causing diarrhoea or constipation can also be alleviated.

respiratory system
The leaf is thought to be more specific for the respiratory system; its mucilaginous quality soothes and acts as an expectorant, making it ideal in the treatment of bronchitis, coughs and sore throats.

genitourinary system
Marshmallow leaf has an affinity with the urinary system, soothing irritation and inflammation and protecting mucous membranes from irritating substances which may be present in the bladder or connecting tubes. It is one of the most effective herbs for alleviating symptoms of cystitis and urethritis.

contraindications
None known.

preparations and dosage
The flowers are not usually available commercially but can be used to make expectorant syrups for coughs.

tea the best way to infuse Marshmallow root is to steep it in cold water for a few hours, or overnight, to get the most demulcent activity from it. Use 1 teaspoon to 1 cup. The leaf can be prepared as a tea using 1 teaspoon per cup, infuse it for 15 minutes and drink freely.

tincture 1 part root or leaf to 5 parts 25% alcohol (white wine). Take 2–5ml in water three times daily.

poultice both root and leaf can be used as a poultice to draw out toxins from the skin, for example when treating boils. Grind the herb into a powder and mix it with water, or an infusion, to create a creamy consistency which is easy to apply to the affected area. Bandage the affected area to hold the poultice in place. Leave it on overnight or as long as necessary and if it dries out replace as required.

combinations

For cystitis the leaf blends well with Cornsilk, Elderflower, Echinacea, Golden rod and Uva ursi. As a soothing expectorant the leaf works well with Elecampane, Thyme and Liquorice. As a treatment for inflammation of the digestive tract and indigestion it can be mixed with Fennel, Chamomile, Lemon balm and Peppermint. As a drawing ointment the powder can be mixed with tincture or tea made from Echinacea to add an antibacterial, blood-purifying element.

meadowsweet

Filipendula ulmaria

parts used
Aerial parts.

collection
The fully-opened flowers and leaves are collected between June and August.

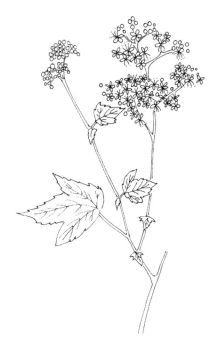

cultivation
This is easy to grow from seed and some varieties are readily available as small plants in garden centres. It prefers a semi-shady position and moisture, so keep the soil well-watered, and perhaps apply a mulch to help retain moisture.

constituents
Salicylic acid, tannin, citric acid, flavonoids, essential oil, and phenolic glycosides

actions
Antacid, anti-rheumatic, stomachic, anti-thrombotic, anti-coagulant, astringent, diaphoretic, diuretic, anti-ulcer, hepatic, anti-inflammatory, mild urinary analgesic.

indications
digestive system
Meadowsweet works in the digestive system to protect mucous membranes by reducing excess acidity. This effect is especially beneficial when treating heartburn, reflux gastritis and gastric or peptic ulcers. It is gently astringent, tones the mucous membranes and is gentle enough to be used to treat diarrhoea in children.

circulatory system
Its role in the circulatory system is due to the presence of salicylic acid, the chemical from which aspirin was first synthesised. It works like aspirin as a mild analgesic and anti-coagulant, and is useful as a preventative to thrombosis but much less likely to cause side effects. However if you are allergic to aspirin, do not risk using Meadowsweet as there is some risk that it could cause the same response.

musculoskeletal system
This is an effective antirheumatic herb due it its aspirin-like, anti-inflammatory action.

urinary system
Meadowsweet is a mild urinary analgesic and antiseptic, worth considering if suffering from a painful bout of cystitis.

contraindications
Allergy to aspirin.

preparations and dosage
tea 2 teaspoons of the dried herb per cup, infuse for 15 minutes and drink three times daily.
tincture 1 part herb to 5 parts 45% alcohol. Take 2–4ml in water three times daily.

combinations
It combines well with Hawthorn and Lime flower in the treatment of high blood pressure. For cystitis mix it with a demulcent such as Cornsilk and an anti-infective such as Uva ursi or Echinacea. When working with arthritis or rheumatism combine it with Celery seed and Ginger. For stomach disorders, like gastritis and heartburn, blend with Chamomile and Marshmallow root.

milk thistle

Carduus marianus

parts used
Seeds.

collection
The mature seed heads are ready for harvesting at the end of the summer. Store them in a warm place and after a few days tap the heads to release the seeds.

cultivation
This large thistle is easy to grow from seed. Sow the seed into open ground in spring and water well. It produces very spiky foliage and flowers so beware when handling the plant as it can be prickly.

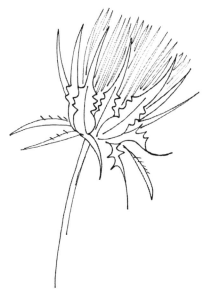

constituents
Silymarin, silychristin, silybin, silydianin, essential oil, bitter principle, mucilage.

actions
Bitter tonic, cholagogue, galactagogue, demulcent, antioxidant, antidepressant, detoxifier, antiviral, liver and gall bladder protector.

indications
digestive system
Milk thistle is well known as a herb for preventing and treating hangovers. It helps to protect the liver from toxins and can be used to prevent cell damage and cirrhosis caused by alcohol, mushroom poisons and environmental toxins. It can also be used to treat the side effects of alcohol and drug addiction, primarily the associated depression and melancholy. It can also assist where there is poor digestion of fats.

genitourinary system
The action milk thistle has on the liver improves its function and, as it improves, the liver is more able to break down and expel

excess hormones thereby relieving pre-menstrual tension caused by hormonal imbalance. Pre-menstrual tension, however, has many causes and associated factors, so it is worth using it in conjunction with other herbs to treat this condition effectively. The tea can also be used to increase breast milk in nursing mothers.

contraindications
None known.

preparations and dosage
decoction half a teaspoon per cup, boil for 15 minutes and drink three times daily.
tincture the tincture can be made up to 1 part herb to 1 part 45% alcohol. Take 1–2 ml in water three times daily.

combinations
To treat poor liver and gall bladder function use with Dandelion root as a decoction. For pre-menstrual tension use as a tincture and blend with Rose, Chamomile or Lemon balm.

motherwort

Leonorus cardiaca

parts used
Aerial parts.

collection
Collect the aerial parts during July and August when flowering.

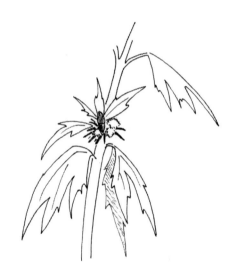

cultivation
Motherwort is very easy to grow and propagates by self-seeding each year. Roots also last a long time in the soil. It is not at all fussy as to the type of soil and is completely hardy.

constituents
Bitter glycosides including Leonurin and leonuridine. Alkoloids including leonuinine and stachydrene, volatile oil and tannin

actions
Sedative, nervine, emmenagogue, antispasmodic, cardiac tonic.

indications
nervous system
This herb works especially well for people who need a big herbal hug for whatever reason. It works to relieve irritability and promote a calm, relaxed and comfortable state of being. It also eases depression, especially that which appears as a symptom of menopause, or pre-menstrual tension. It is also useful for insomnia and general nervousness.

genitourinary system
Used to relieve period pains, and regulate periods.

circulatory system
A tonic for the heart, especially where weakness has been caused by nervous debility, and helps in the treatment of palpitations. It is also a hypotensive, normalising high blood pressure.

contraindications
None known.

preparations and dosage
tea use 1–2 teaspoons per cup, infuse for 10 minutes and drink three times daily.

tincture 1 part herb to 5 parts 45% alcohol, infuse for 2 weeks and macerate daily. Take 5ml in water three times daily.

combinations
When treating insomnia combine with Passionflower and Lime flower. This herb can be used to treat stress-related high blood pressure combined with a mild diuretic, such as Dandelion leaf, and another relaxing vasodilator, such as Lime flower.

myrrh

Commiphora molmol

parts used
Resin. I recommend always using commercially produced products for Myrrh as it is very difficult to work with.

collection
Myrrh is available as an essential oil, as peas or as powder (see supplier details Page 162). It is a tree which grows in the deserts of North Africa. The resin is still collected in a traditional manner by nomadic people and sold on for distribution throughout the world.

cultivation

A tree normally found in deserts and not suitable for cultivation in Britain without specialist facilities.

constituents

Essential oil, resin, gums

actions

Antiviral, anti-bacterial, anti-microbial, increases white blood cell count in the blood, astringent, anti-catarrhal, expectorant, vulnerary.

indications

skin

The essential oil, the tincture and the resin can all be used topically on the skin to heal and anti-infect almost any wound. The astringent, binding effect helps to heal skin fast; it seems to create its own scab, drying across the wound and then tightening up, pulling the edges of the wound together whilst treating and protecting from infection.

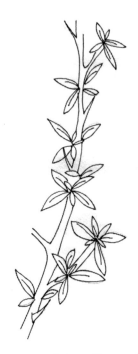

respiratory system

Myrrh can be used internally as a tincture or externally as an essential oil to treat infections of the lungs and if the body's immune system needs a boost. It is particularly of benefit for respiratory infections as it has expectorant and anticatarrhal properties, relieving the symptoms associated with colds and flu.

contraindications

Do not use during pregnancy.

preparations and dosage

tincture take 2–3ml three times daily in water. The tincture is 90% alcohol, so please *always* dilute in water before using internally.

essential oil to use topically on a small clean wound, apply neat (the tincture can also be used in this way). To add to a chest rub use 1–2%, up to 36 drops in 60ml base.

combinations

As a chest rub for a respiratory infection it blends well with Rosemary, Peppermint, Eucalyptus or Tea tree essential oils.

Internally as a tincture for respiratory conditions blend with Echinacea, Sage and Marshmallow root. You can also add the tincture to a tea for this purpose.

peppermint

Mentha x piperita

parts used
Aerial parts.

collection
The aerial parts should be collected on a dry day just before the flowers open. The stems are then tied together loosely into bunches and hung to dry. When dry place in an airtight container to prevent re-absorption of moisture.

cultivation
Peppermint is very easy to grow from seed planted in the spring. Different varieties are available from garden centres. It can be invasive so be prepared to chop it back hard in the summer.

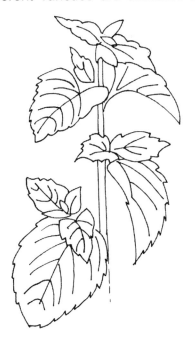

constituents
The plant contains up to 2% essential oil containing tannins, menthol. Other constituents include menthone, jasmine, bitter principle, flavanoids.

actions
Carminative, antispasmodic, analgesic, nervine, antiseptic diaphoretic, aromatic, anti-emetic, antiseptic, source of potassium and magnesium, emmenagogue and enzyme activator,.

indications
digestive system
Peppermint has a great affinity with the digestive system and, as a carminative, antispasmodic and digestive juice and bile secretion

stimulant; it can be used to treat indigestion, travel sickness, flatulence and colic. The essential oil acts as a mild anaesthetic to the stomach wall and allays feelings of nausea and the desire to vomit.

respiratory system
Peppermint is a cooling diaphoretic and useful for treating fevers associated with any type of infection, whether respiratory, digestive or urinary. This is especially useful when treating infants who have had a high fever causing febrile convulsions. Please note, however, that the essential oil is contraindicated in epilepsy as it is a mild neurotoxin in high doses due to its menthone content. The tea is safe, just avoid the oil for children, in high doses or for epileptics.

genitourinary system
It can be used as an antispasmodic to relieve painful period cramps and the associated emotional tension.

skin
Externally it can be used as a mild anaesthetic to relieve itching and is good to treat a hot eczema. It is best to use the essential oil blended at a 0.5% maximum dilution.

contraindications
Pregnancy.

preparations and dosage
tea 2 teaspoons per cup, infuse for 10 minutes and drink freely.
tincture 1 part peppermint to 5 parts 45% alcohol. Take 2–4ml in water daily.
inhalation 1 drop of oil in a bowl of steaming water. Inhale the steam for 5 minutes to treat headaches, colds and mental exhaustion.
essential oil to make a massage oil use 5–6 drops in 2 teaspoons of oil for cramps, spasms, muscular pains, lower back ache and stiff joints
cream the essential oil can also be added to a base cream for use on hot skin conditions such as eczema, but be careful as it may cause irritation if the person has sensitive skin.

combinations
For fevers blend Peppermint with Elderflower and Yarrow. For digestive problems it works well with Chamomile and Marshmallow root.

plantain

Plantago lanceolata, Plantago majoralis

parts used
Leaves.

collection
Collect the leaves any time throughout the summer and dry as quickly as possible to prevent a loss of coloration.

cultivation
Plantain, like dandelion, is generally considered to be a weed, which invades lawns and is found in most grassy areas. It is not something I have ever had to cultivate!

constituents
Flavonoids, tannins, iridoids, mucilage, glycosides.

actions
Expectorant, demulcent, astringent, diuretic, anti-histamine, anti-bacterial, anti-allergy, blood tonic, lymphatic, anti-haemorrhagic, anti-acid (tea).

indications
respiratory system

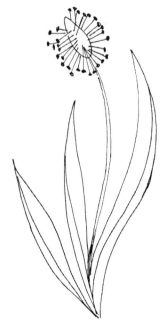

Its gentle, expectorant and soothing demulcent actions help to ease dry coughs. The anti-histamine and anti-allergy action eases the congestion and inflammation caused by hayfever and other allergies affecting the respiratory tract. It is also quite specific for inflammation of the eustachian tube causing earache and I have not yet found another herb quite as good at relieving this pain.

digestive system
Its strong demulcent activity works wonders to soothe an irritated or inflamed digestive system, while its astringent properties can prove useful for treating haemorrhoids and diarrhoea.

urinary system
As an antibacterial, diuretic and demulcent this is a good herb to choose for cystitis.

contraindications
None known.

preparations and dosage
tea 2 teaspoons of dried herb per cup, or 3 of the fresh herb, infuse for 15 minutes and drink freely.
tincture 1 part herb to 5 parts 25% alcohol. Take 5–10ml in water daily.

combinations
For hayfever and sinusitis make a tea with Peppermint, Elderflower, Eyebright, and Nettle or Chamomile. As a remedy for coughs and bronchitis add to Thyme and Elecampane. To treat an inflamed or infected urinary system use it blended with Echinacea, Uva ursi and Calendula.

raspberry

Rubus idaeus

parts used
Leaves.

collection
The leaves may be collected throughout the growing season. Dry slowly in a well-ventilated area to ensure proper preservation of the properties.

cultivation
This is a great herb to grow as you get to enjoy the raspberries too. The bramble is easy to find as small plants at garden centres and can be grown against a fence.

constituents
Tannins, polypeptides, flavonoids.

actions
Pre-natal aid, astringent tonic, antispasmodic, parturient with a reputation for painless and easy delivery in straightforward births.

indications
genitourinary system
Raspberry leaf has a long tradition of use in pregnancy to strengthen and tone the tissue of the womb, assisting contractions

and checking any haemorrhage during labour. To get the best effect from this herb the tea needs to be drunk throughout the last six months of pregnancy and during labour. It acts as a general tonic to the reproductive organs of both men and women, encouraging healthy circulation to the reproductive system. This action is helpful where impotence in men is caused by reduced blood flow due to poor health and it encourages better health of the prostate gland by aiding circulation to the area. In women it works to regulate the menstrual cycle and, as an antispasmodic, it can relieve the cramping associated with painful periods.

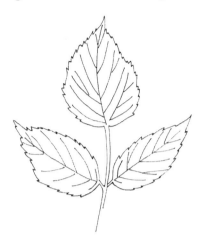

digestive system
Raspberry leaf can be used as an astringent mouthwash to treat mouth ulcers.

contraindications
Some sources contraindicate Raspberry leaf during the first trimester of pregnancy.

preparations and dosage
tea use 1–3 teaspoons per cup, infuse for 10–15 minutes, drink three cups daily.
tincture 1 part herb to 5 parts 25% alcohol. Take 5 ml in water three times daily.

combinations
For painful periods it works well with Motherwort, Cramp bark and Valerian. For heavy bleeding it can be used with Yarrow and Ladies mantle. For impotence caused by lack of circulation try it with Ginkgo and Damiana.

rose

Rosa damascena, Rosa gallica, Rosa centifolia

parts used
Petals.

collection

Collect the petals from the flower in full bloom on a dry day, dry them in a dark area to retain the colour and fairly gently: an airing cupboard makes an ideal spot for this.

cultivation

Three varieties are grown for herbal medicine: Rosa damascena, gallica and centifolia. They may take a little finding as they are not the most popular varieties and aren't always available in garden

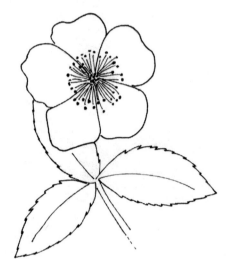

centres, but they are all are native to northern Europe so will grow happily in Britain in manure-enriched soil in full sun.

constituents

Essential oil containing nerol, geraniol, eugenol.

actions

Mild sedative, mild local anaesthetic, cooling skin astringent, anti-inflammatory, liver protector, aphrodisiac, anti-depressant, cardioactive, cholagogue, antispasmodic, antiviral, menstrual regulator.

indications
genitourinary system

Rose has a regulatory function on the menstrual cycle, and also works to alleviate emotional tension associated with premenstrual tension via its action on both the liver and the nervous system. As an antispasmodic it also works to reduce muscle spasm associated with painful periods.

skin

The essential oil and aromatic water can be used as topical applications, to reduce inflammation and redness. It also has some action on thread veins which appear on the face with age, sunburn, or alcohol use.

nervous system

Rose is a fantastic antidepressant used in any of its available forms. It works to heal our broken hearts from anger, loss and grief, helping us to love ourselves and others again. Perhaps this is why lovers give each other roses. It also works to calm an anxious heart and prevent panic attacks and the associated palpitations.

digestive system
Rose works within the digestive system primarily as a liver protector and cholagogue. It is not as strong as Milk thistle in its action but can be of benefit nevertheless.

contraindications
None known

preparations and dosage
tea 1–2 teaspoons of fresh or dried flowers per cup, infuse for 10 minutes and drink freely.

tincture 1 part herb to 1 part 45% alcohol. Take 2ml in water three times daily.

aromatic water for internal take use 5ml three times daily. On the skin, use freely.

essential oil Rose oil is generally very expensive, about 60p per drop in its pure form, and, as a result, is usually sold in an adulterated form. It is worth finding a reputable source if you wish to use the oil for medicinal purposes rather than just for its scent.

combinations
For regulating the menstrual cycle use with Raspberry leaf. As an antidepressant use with Lemon balm.

rosemary
Rosmarinus officinalis

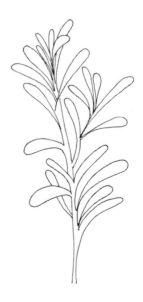

parts used
Leaves and terminal twigs.

collection
The leaves can be gathered throughout the growing season but they are at their best while they are flowering in April and May. Dry in a dark, not too warm, area to prevent loss of the essential oil component.

cultivation
Propagate from cuttings or buy small plants to grow on from garden centres. It is very easy to grow but

prefers a sunny, sheltered position with good drainage.

constituents

Essential oil, cineole, linalol, camphene, camphor, tannins, bitter principle, diterpenes, flavonoids.

actions

Nervine, antispasmodic, antidepressive, antiseptic, rubefacient, circulatory tonic.

indications

musculoskeletal system

Rosemary acts topically as a rubefacient oil, improving circulation and the healing of sprains and strains. It can work to release muscle tension, especially if used in a massage as an infused or essential oil.

nervous system

It improves memory and, as a result of its action on the liver, can ease headaches associated with digestive problems or toxicity. It also acts as a nervine and antispasmodic and as such can ease headaches caused by tension leading to poor circulation in the shoulders. Its action as a nervine is quite energising, relieving tiredness and feelings of melancholic-type depression, restoring motivation and clear thinking.

circulatory system

Rosemary is a gentle circulatory stimulant and improves circulation specifically to the head. It is a traditional herb for maintaining a healthy head of hair, used internally, and externally as a hair rinse. It can also be of use to help postural hypertension: the feeling of dizziness when getting up from sitting or lying down.

contraindications

None known.

preparations and dosage

tea 1 teaspoon per cup, infuse for 10 minutes and drink three cups daily.

tincture 1 part herb to 5 parts 45% alcohol. Take 2–4ml in water three times daily.

rosemary wine infuse 30g of freshly picked, terminal shoots, in white wine for 1 week, decant, strain and store in the fridge. Take half to 1 wine glass full daily.

essential oil use 10 drops per 30ml base oil and massage into painful or aching muscles and joints.

combinations

For dizziness mix with Hawthorn and Ginger. As an antidepressant it works well with St. John's wort and Lemon balm. As a massage ointment for muscle aches, strains and sprains mix the essential oil of Rosemary and Ginger or Juniper in a base of Arnica ointment or in a base oil, using a maximum of 10 drops in 30g of base.

sage, greek sage

Salvia officinalis, Salvia triloba

parts used

Leaves.

collection

The leaves should be gathered shortly before, or just at the beginning of, flowering in dry, sunny weather during May or June. Dry in the shade and not above 35°C.

cultivation

This herb grows wild in the warmer parts of the Mediterranean and prefers similar growing conditions, ideally a warm sunny spot with good soil. It is easy to grow either from seed or readily available in garden centres. Sow outside in spring and thin out to encourage healthy plants. The sage tends to get a bit leggy after three years growth so it may be necessary to replace the plant every few years to keep it looking fresh.

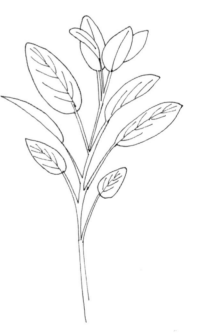

constituents

sage essential oil including 30% thujone, 5% cineole, linalol, borneol, camphor, salvene and pinene, bitter principle, tannins, triterpenoids, flavonoids, oestrogenic substances, resin.

greek sage there are significantly lower levels of thujone, which can be neurotoxic if used in excess, in this than in other varieties of sage, so this is the safest to use internally. Also linalol, borneol, camphor, salvene and pinene, bitter principle, tannins, triterpenoids, flavonoids, oestrogenic substances, resin.

actions
Carminative, antispasmodic, antiseptic, astringent, antibiotic, circulatory stimulant (especially to the head), diaphoretic, associated with wisdom and longevity in folk medicine.

indications
respiratory system
Sage is one of the best remedies for a sore throat, inflamed glands and tonsils and general inflammation of the mucous membranes in the mouth. It works as an antibiotic and anti-infective to treat the infection causing the problem and also soothes the membranes directly. As a diaphoretic it is useful in fevers often associated with respiratory infections.

genitourinary system
This herb is also well known for its so called oestrogenic activity in menopause and, although research suggests there are no chemicals found in sage which can be responsible for this action, it is still the best herb for reducing hot flushes and night sweats, even if we can't explain how it works just yet.

digestive system
As an antispasmodic carminative it is useful for treating wind and irritable bowel syndrome.

cardiovascular system
As a circulatory tonic it has an action on the head, aids memory and can help to reduce mental confusion.

contraindications
As Sage stimulates the muscles of the uterus it should be avoided during pregnancy. Due to its high thujone and camphor content, both can be neurotoxic in excess, it should also be avoided in large quantities and not taken for an extended period.

preparations and dosage
tea use 1–2 teaspoons per cup and drink three times daily.
tincture Take 1 ml in water three times daily.
essential oil has a very high thujone content and is best avoided.

combinations

To use as a mouth wash or gargle for a sore throat mix in equal parts with Marigold, Echinacea and Myrrh. Dilute the tinctures, using 5ml tincture to a quarter of a cup of water, swill, gargle and spit. As a tonic to the brain and to improve memory blend with Gingko and Rosemary.

st. john's wort

Hypericum perforatum

parts used

Aerial parts when in flower, at the end of June.

collection

The entire plant above ground is used and collected when in flower, and dried as quickly as possible.

cultivation

Easy to grow from seed and from divided root stock.

constituents

Rutin, essential oil, tannin, resin, pectin, hypericins.

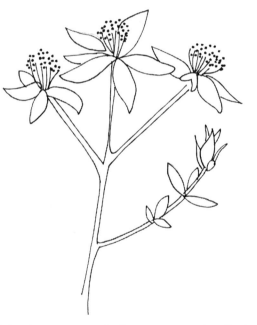

actions

Alterative, antidepressant, antiviral, relaxing nervine, sedative, anti-inflammatory, astringent, vulnerary.

indications
nervous system

St. John's wort is a relaxing tonic for the nervous system and is of benefit where any trauma, shock or long-term depression or anxiety has caused the person to feel emotionally debilitated. It is especially useful in menopausal depression. It also works as a mild analgesic and anti-inflammatory and is very effective for treating sciatica, facial neuralgia, loss of sensation and tingling sensations in the periphery of the body.

skin
Topically St. John' wort infused oil is useful as a mild analgesic for nerve pain and as a vulnerary for wounds which are painful or difficult to heal, such as burns and animal bites.

contraindications
Do not take this herb internally if you are having medication for heart problems, depression, mental illness, epilepsy or taking the contraceptive pill, as St. John's wort may cause the body to improve its liver function and thereby break down these prescriptive drugs more quickly, reducing their efficacy.

preparations and dosage
tea 2 teaspoons per cup, infuse for 15 minutes and drink three times daily.

tincture 1 part herb to 10 parts 45% alcohol. Take 2–4ml in water three times daily.

infused oil collect the open flowers, add them to a base oil, leave in the sun for three weeks and strain. Use topically as required.

combinations
For menopausal anxiety, fatigue and depression it combines well with Motherwort, Rosemary and Sage. To treat depression blend with Rosemary, Lemon balm and Oat straw. As a massage oil to treat nerve pain add Lavender essential oil at 1% dilution, 9 drops in 30ml oil.

skullcap

Scutelaria laterifolia

parts used
Aerial parts.

collection
Aerial parts can be collected whilst flowering during August and September.

cultivation
This herb is happy in any garden in a sunny position .The plants only last for two or three years so cultivation is best continued by collecting seed. Use a hot bed to promote germination in March then plant straight into open soil in April.

constituents
Flavonoid glycosides, including scutellarian and scutellarein; trace of essential oil, bitter, tannin, fat, sugar and cellulose.

actions
Tonic, sedative. nervine, antispasmodic, astringent,

indications
nervous system
This is one of the best herbs for treating insomnia and the nervous system in general. It helps to calm an anxious mind, reducing the number and speed of thoughts that often flood the mind during times of anxiety and episodes of insomnia. I have had great results with this herb in cases of addiction and obsessive compulsive disorder. Skullcap seems to really help where obsessive thoughts are hard to switch off or tone down,.

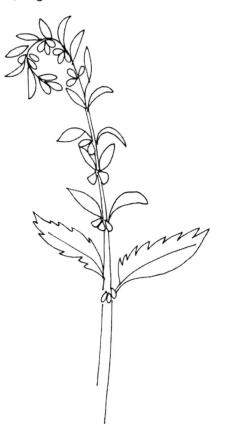

contraindications
Large doses may cause giddiness so keep to recommended doses.

preparations and dosage
tea use 1–2 teaspoons per cup, infuse for 10 minutes and drink three times daily.

tincture 1 part herb to 5 parts 45% alcohol, infuse for 2 weeks and macerate daily. Take 5ml in water three times daily.

combinations
Fantastic with Chamomile, Lime flower or Valerian, or any number of nervine herbs, to promote emotional wellbeing and relaxation.

thyme

Thymus vulgaris

parts used
Dried leaves and flowering tops.

collection
The flowering branches are collected between June and August on a dry, sunny day. Dry the branches then strip the leaves and flowers off and store in an airtight container.

cultivation
Thyme is not easy to grow from seed. Many varieties exist and can be found in most garden centres as small plants. It enjoys full sun in a rich well-drained compost and will be very happy in a pot on the patio.

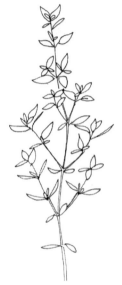

constituents
Thymol, carvacrol, thymol, linalol, borneol, bitter principles, tannin, flavonoids, triterpenoids.

actions
Carminative, anti-microbial, anti-spasmodic, diuretic, expectorant, antitussive, astringent, anthelmintic, antifungal, anti-oxidant, antiseptic.

indications
respiratory system
Thyme's action as an antimicrobial, antitussive, expectorant makes it a powerful remedy for all coughs and chest infections. It is active against viral and bacterial infections and has a gentle warming action helping to push out those chilly feelings associated with sore throats, flu, colds and bronchitis, especially in the winter time.

digestive system
It is an anthelmintic: garden Thyme is known to be active against hookworm. As an antispasmodic and carminative for the digestive system it is a good herb for dyspepsia and sluggish digestion.

genitourinary system

Its antimicrobial action is of most use in treating this system of the body as it is active against the pathogens which cause thrush and cystitis. It is most effective used as a tea but it is too hot a herb to use as a douche or to add to the bath.

contraindications

None known.

preparations and dosage

tea half to 1 teaspoon per cup, infuse for 15 minutes. Drink three times daily, or every hour in acute cases.

tincture 1 part herb to 5 parts 45% alcohol, macerate for 8 days and strain. Take 30–60 drops in water three times daily.

combinations

For chesty coughs use it with a soothing demulcent such as Marshmallow leaf and an immune enhancer such as Echinacea. For a sore throat use with lymphatic tonics such as Calendula and another astringent like Sage or Myrrh. Echinacea can also be added for its numbing action when gargled. In treating cystitis it blends well with Marshmallow and Cornsilk.

valerian

Valerian officinalis

parts used

Rhizome and root.

collection

Collect the roots in late autumn, clean them thoroughly and dry in the shade. Keep them away from cats as they love the smell and will eat them if given the opportunity.

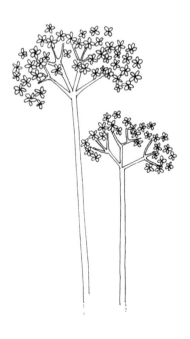

cultivation

Valerian is tolerant of most soil types in sun or shade. Propagate by sowing the seed in spring. Cutting off the flowers will encourage a larger rhizome for harvesting.

constituents
Essential oil, valerianic acid, isovalerianic acid, borneol, pinene, camphene, alkaloids, valepotriates.

actions
Sedative, hypnotic, anti-spasmodic, hypotensive, carminative, mild anodyne for temporary relief of pain, relaxant.

indications

nervous system
Valerian acts to calm both the central and peripheral nervous system, relaxing the mind and the body. This action helps it to relieve pain and act as an anti-stress medicine. It also has the ability to lower high blood pressure, especially where it is stress related. It is the number one remedy for difficulty with sleeping, whether you can't get off to sleep or find it hard to sleep through the night. Valerian seems to take the edge of the harshness of reality when things just get too much. It works like the tranquilliser Valium on the GABA receptors within the brain but does not have the side effects of Valium or carry the risk of addiction. If you attempt an overdose, for instance, the only side effect will be that you feel sleepy for a short while.

cardiovascular system
Its antispasmodic effect on the body also affects the muscles in the arterioles and arteries and this effect, with its relaxant quality, enables it to lower high blood pressure. It is also a good herb for anxiety, palpitations, and panic attacks.

digestive system
Valerian is mildly bitter, encouraging the release of digestive juices and healthy digestion. As an antispasmodic it relaxes the cramps associated with colic and wind.

contraindications
Very rarely Valerian has a stimulating effect on some people. This is only mild but if it happens discontinue use immediately and look for an alternative. As Valerian is a sedative do not take large doses of it before driving or operating machinery.

preparations and dosage
tea half to 1 teaspoon per cup, infuse for 15 minutes and drink three times daily.
tincture 1 part root to 5 parts 45% alcohol. Take 1–3 in water three times daily.

combinations

For relief of period pains, or other cramping pains, combine with Cramp bark and Ginger. As this tastes pretty disgusting as a tea, I would advise taking it in tincture form. To encourage a good night's sleep blend with Passionflower and Chamomile. To treat high blood pressure blend with Yarrow, Lime flower and Hawthorn but be aware that if the person is on medication they must seek advice from a health professional before combining herbs and orthodox medications as they can interact.

vervain

Verbena officinalis

parts used
Aerial flowering parts.

collection
Collect this herb just before it opens its flowers, which is usually in July.

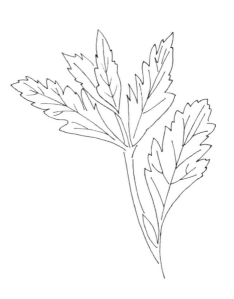

cultivation
Vervain is easy to grow in anything from semi-shade to full sun. It is easy to find from an herb specialist or herb farm and has lovely purple flowers in late summer.

constituents
Alkaloids, bitter glycosides called verbanalin, essential oil, mucilage, tannin, flavanoids.

actions
Astringent, diaphoretic, antispasmodic, nervine, sedative, hepatic, galactagogue, aphrodisiac, tonic, anti-diarrhoeic, emmenagogue.

indications
nervous system
A strengthening yet relaxing nervine tonic which helps the mind to become more grounded and focused. It can ease the melancholic type of depression especially where this follows another illness like flu.

digestive system
Used as a hepatic to promote liver function, which would be beneficial in cases of hepatitis and jaundice.

genitourinary system
It is a good general tonic for the reproductive organs, to regulate periods and for the relief of period pain and pre-menstrual tension.

contraindications
None found.

preparations and dosage
tea use 1–2 teaspoons per cup, infuse for 10 minutes and drink three times daily.

tincture 1 part herb to 5 parts 45% alcohol, infuse for 2 weeks and macerate daily. Take 2–4 ml in water three times daily.

combinations
For depression following an illness blend with oats and Echinacea. As an aphrodisiac combine with Damiana and Rose.

yarrow

Achillea millefolium

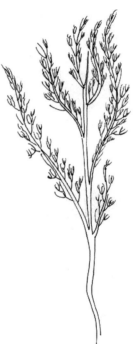

parts used
Aerial parts, flowers and leaves.

collection
The whole of the plant above ground should be collected between June and September when it is in flower.

cultivation
This is another plant commonly found in our lawns and seen as a weed. It is also grown as an ornamental herb in pink and red and white varieties. It is easy to grow from seed sown in the spring and is tolerant of most soil types, full sun and shady positions.

constituents
Flavonoids, volatile oil, sesquiterpene lactones, plant acids, alkaloids, essential oil.

actions

Diaphoretic, anti-inflammatory, antispasmodic, haemostatic, antipyretic, anti-rheumatic, choleretic, bitter, diuretic, antiseptic, urinary antiseptic, hypotensive, carminative, digestive tonic, emmenagogue, a gentle relaxant like Chamomile.

indications

respiratory system

Yarrow is one of the best diaphoretic herbs and can be used for temperature reduction in fever, influenza, colds and other feverish complaints and is particularly useful for children.

circulatory system

It normalises blood flow and stems inappropriate blood flow so is useful for treating nosebleeds. It acts to improve overall circulation, lowering blood pressure by improving peripheral circulation and can also be useful in treating high blood pressure associated with thrombosis.

digestive system

Yarrow has an antispasmodic action on stomach cramps and acts as a gentle tonic for the digestion. Its carminative action relieves bloating by helping to expel wind. It also improves liver and gall bladder function as a choleretic, helping the release of bile for digestion.

genitourinary system

As a normaliser of blood flow it helps to stem excess blood flow in menorrhagia but also helps to bring on a period where it is delayed. As an antispasmodic it relieves cramping period pain and is used as a urinary antiseptic to treat cystitis.

musculoskeletal system

Yarrow is antirheumatic which is probably due to its overall action in improving digestion and elimination, and also reducing inflammation and spasm.

contraindications

Very large doses may cause headache.

preparations and dosage

tea use 1 teaspoon per cup and infuse for 15 minutes. When feverish this tea can be drunk every hour.

fresh juice extract from leaves and flowers and take half to 1 teaspoon.

tincture 1 part herb to 5 parts 25% alcohol. Take 1–2 ml in water up to three times daily.

bath to relieve rheumatic pain, inflammation of joints or muscles, and muscle spasm, infuse 25g herb in 2 litres of water for 10 minutes, strain and add to the bath.

essential oil apply at 0.5–1% dilution added to a base oil, cream or gel to ease inflammation and cramping pain.

combinations

For raised blood pressure it can be combined with Hawthorn flowers and Lime flower. For fevers it combines well with Peppermint, Elderflower, Boneset and Lime flower.

how to make herbal medicines

This is where we get really practical and show you how to make your own herbal medicine preparations, from teas to creams and ointments, from wines to herbal honeys. There are several recipes for each type of preparation that can be made at home without too much technical experience or specialist equipment required. They can be followed to the letter or be used as a basis for your own creative flair. Most importantly this practical part of the book has been devised to help you gain in confidence, guiding you step-by step so you can learn to utilise herbs in a way which is suitable for your needs. Enjoy!

blending herb teas

Herbs can be blended harmoniously to produce a mix which works better than a single herb, or simply tastes better. Peppermint is useful to add to the bitterer herbs, such as Yarrow, as it will help to improve the flavour, or Liquorice can be added for those with a sweet tooth.

Blending to get the right taste is a personal thing and trial and error is the best way to learn: – there are no rules to ensure success.

When blending for medicinal effect chose herbs that are working towards the same effect. Keep it simple and don't try to treat lots of complaints all at once or you will end up diluting the effect. Keeping the blend simple allows you to analyse the effect of the tea and perhaps change it if necessary. You can blend herbs in equal parts or have more of one than another. Taste and medicinal action can guide your decision.

A good example would be a herb tea for high blood pressure. Think about the actions you need to help lower the blood pressure. These are helping peripheral circulation and relaxing mind and body. There are many herbs which work in this way and you could choose to blend two to four of them together, perhaps

Yarrow, Lime flower, Hawthorn and Motherwort. If the person you are blending the tea for would prefer the tea to taste less bitter you could replace one of the herbs with Peppermint to improve the taste.

The overall amount of herb to use per cup, whether singly or blended, varies depending on how bulky or finely chopped the herb is. Once again a combination of taste and medicinal requirements govern how much you should use. The general rule is 2 teaspoons per cup, brew for 15 minutes, strain and drink up to three cups daily.

The teas can be drunk warm, cool or iced and last up to twenty-four hours if kept in a fridge.

detox tea
Marigold flowers
Peppermint
Elderflower
Cleavers
Blend in equal parts, use 2–3 teaspoons per cup, drink three cups daily.

relax tea
Lime flower
Chamomile
Lemon balm
Passionflower
Blend in equal parts using 2–3 teaspoons per cup. Drink three cups daily.

blending decoctions

Decoctions are required when extracting the medicinal chemicals from the tougher parts of a plant: the roots, bark and berries. Flavour isn't something one needs to consider here as decoctions never taste delicious. As a general rule the dosage is 2 teaspoons per cup, starting with a cup and a half of water, as some will evaporate and be absorbed by the plant material during the boiling process. The plant matter and water are brought to the boil and simmered for 20 minutes, then strained. The softer parts of the plant can be added to a decoction mix once it has been boiled. They should be left to infuse in the boiled solution for a further 10 minutes before straining. One cup of decoction will give you two or three doses which can be spread out over a day.

Decoctions last up to 3 days in a fridge and alcohol or honey can be added to preserve them. Add 450g honey to 200ml of decoction. Take 1 teaspoon of the blended honey and decoction mix three times daily.

Add spirits at a ratio of 1 part spirit to 2 parts decoction (for 45% alcohol use vodka), the maximum dose should be 15ml twice daily and watch the alcohol content if driving!

liver healing decoction
Dandelion root
Milk thistle seed
Use equal parts of the herbs, simmer for 20 minutes, strain, allow to cool a little and drink.

antispasmodic decoction
Valerian root   1 part
Cramp bark   3 parts
Ginger root   1 part
Simmer for 20 minutes, strain, allow to cool a little and drink.

tinctures

Tinctures are the alcoholic extract of the herb and can be made at various strengths using 25% to 90% alcohol. The highest percentage alcohol available, unless you have a Customs and Excise alcohol licence for medicine making, is 45% and vodka is most commonly used although other spirits can be employed. The usual ratio of herb to alcohol is 1:5, which means, for example, 10g of plant matter to 50ml alcohol although this ratio can vary from 2:1 to 1:20 depending on the strength of the herb and the purpose of the tincture being made. The guidelines followed by most herbalists come from the *British Herbal Pharmacopoeia* (see Page 166).

Use the following method to make tinctures:

Chop or bruise the fresh or dried herb.

Put the herb into a jar and add the alcohol.

Leave to stand in a cool, dark place for 2 weeks and shake the jar daily.

Strain the tincture through a piece of fabric or muslin, squeeze the herb to extract every drop of liquid. then discard the used herb.

Pour this liquid into a clean glass bottle or jar for storage. A dark-coloured container is best. If using plastic bottles make sure they are food grade and will not interact with the alcohol.

There are other types of tinctures made in a very similar way which are available to medical herbalists. These are called distilled, infused, and decocted tinctures. They are made by the same method but some of the volume of liquid is substituted with an infusion, decoction or the aromatic water. These types of tincture are much stronger and are currently only readily available to medical herbalists, although they are not restricted for sale to the public and you can make them yourself.

vinegar extracts

Traditionally cider vinegar and wine vinegars have been used to produce herbal medicines throughout Europe. They are better for people who do not tolerate alcohol well. Cider vinegar, additionally, has its own medicinal benefit.

Medicinal vinegars are made in exactly the same way as tinctures. Follow the step-by-step guide and simply replace the alcohol with vinegar. Cider vinegar and wine vinegar are better than malt vinegar as their flavours are more delicate.

herbal honeys

Honey is the best preservative on the planet; it lasts forever and is highly anti-microbial, protecting anything in it from going mouldy or oxidising. It is also delicious and a very good way of getting medicines into fussy children. It can be added to decoctions for internal use (see Page 132) and to herb juices. Garlic juice added to honey is especially good as a poultice for cuts, grazes and other small skin wounds.

honey based syrup

Honey can be used to make syrups too as follows:

Chop 40g of fresh herb, add 900ml of water, place the ingredients into a saucepan, bring to the boil, cover and simmer for 20 minutes.

Allow the liquid to cool and strain into a measuring jug, pressing all the liquid out of the herb.

Return this liquid to the heat and simmer gently, uncovered to reduce the volume to approximately 200ml.

Keeping the saucepan on the heat add 450ml of honey and allow it to dissolve into the liquid until the consistency is syrupy. Be careful not to overheat it, as this will cause the texture to become like toffee. Pour this syrup into a clean container and store in a cool, dark place.

Dosage for adults: 2–3 teaspoons, three times daily.

Dosage for children: 1 teaspoon, 3–6 times daily.

capsules

When choosing a blend of herbs for a capsule you can concentrate purely on how you want the product to work medicinally. You are not restricted by taste as you may be in blending a tea, or by which parts of a herb you can use. However, I would advise that you keep it simple, and use a blend which is working on just one or two health issues to ensure a higher success rate.

A coffee grinder works well for grinding the herbs but be aware that some of the more fibrous herbs may prove difficult to turn into powder. Using a fine sieve once they are ground can be helpful to extract the powder and leave the fibrous element behind.

It is possible to fill capsules by hand but using a capsule maker allows you to increase the dosage, up to four times higher in some cases, as you can pack a lot more herb into each capsule. There are suppliers listed at the back of the book (see Page 164) if this is something you would like to try.

happy capsules

To treat depression, pre-menstrual tension, melancholy and sadness

Rosemary
St. Johns wort
Lemon balm
Oat straw
Use equal parts of each of the herbs, powdered and well blended.
If a capsule maker is used the average contents of one capsule
will be 350–400mg.
Adult dose: 2 capsules twice daily.

sleepy time capsules
to aid sleep
Valerian
Passionflower
Skullcap
Use equal parts of each of the herbs, powdered and well blended.
If a capsule maker is used the average contents of one capsule
will be 350–400mg.
Adult dose: 2 capsules twice daily.

wines and beers

Herbs can be used as the basis for the fermentation, for example
Elderflower, Elderberry, Hawthorn berry, Rosehip, Dandelion and
Marigold. I am not going into the details of winemaking but would
encourage you to give it a try. There are plenty of introductory
books available and, once you have mastered the essential
process, you can experiment with your own recipes.

Herbs can be also be added to wines, ciders or beers also in a
way that's similar to making a tincture. Aromatic herbs such as
Rosemary, Sage, Thyme, Clove, Cardamom, Cinnamon, Orange
or Juniper are particularly pleasant to add to wines as they have
such strong flavours.

hot spicy cider
A favourite for Guy Fawkes night to help you keep warm.
1 litre of cider. Reasonable quality, traditional English varieties
work best.
6 cloves
4 cinnamon sticks or 4 teaspoons of powder
1 inch of root ginger, chopped

1 tablespoon of honey

Blend all the ingredients together and infuse for 2 weeks. Heat in a covered pan until just boiling then turn off the heat, cooling a little before straining, then drink whilst still warm, or put in a thermos flask to keep warm until required.

uplifting tonic wine
1 bottle of white wine, reasonable quality
1 sprig of fresh thyme
1 sprig of Rosemary
6 Cardamom pods, crushed

Blend all the ingredients together in a suitable container and leave covered for two weeks in an airtight, preferably glass, container. Strain, pour back into the wine bottle and store in a cool dark place.

Adult dose: half a small wine glass full when you require a mentally and physically uplifting tonic.

I use a good German Riesling to make this wine as its sweetness helps to buffer any bitter element extracted from the herbs.

infused oils

Infused oils are made in the same way as tinctures, except oil is used instead of alcohol. They are very easy to prepare and can be used as the basic ingredient of other products such as ointments and creams.

There are no hard and fast rules about the proportions of herb to oil but the tradition is to fill the container with herb so there is an inch left at the top. The herb material should be packed in but not too tightly, that way the oil can coat the herb and extract its medicinal qualities. The size of the container is not important, it just depends on how much infused oil you want to make. Do ensure, if the container is plastic, that it is food grade so the oil and plastic do not interact. Cover the herb with a good quality vegetable oil, I prefer to use organic sunflower or olive oil. The oil should completely cover the herb, leaving about 1cm of oil clear at the top to ensure there is no air penetrating the mix. If it does it will oxidise and go rancid. Also check the 'use by' date of the oil.

This will be the use by date of your infused oil product and should be clearly written on the product's label.

comfrey infused oil
Pick fresh Comfrey leaves on a dry day. Remove any damaged parts or insects. Chop finely. Cover the chopped leaves with an oil of your choice. Leave for two weeks, in a warm, dry place and shake the mixture daily. After the two weeks strain through a piece of muslin and squeeze the herb so every last drop of oil is extracted. Label the container carefully with the 'use by' date of the oil and store in a cool, dark place.

St. John's wort infused oil
Pick the flowers of the plant when in full bloom. Remove any damaged parts or insects. Cover the flowers with an oil of your choice. Leave in a sunny, dry place for two weeks, and shake the mixture daily. The light from the sun causes a chemical reaction in the infusion to produce the red-coloured chemical which works as a pain-relieving anti-inflammatory. After two weeks strain through a piece of muslin and squeeze the herb so every last drop of oil is extracted. Label the container carefully with the 'use by' date of the oil and store in a cool, dark place.

hot oil
Warming, antispasmodic oil
This is a slightly different method of making an infused oil using heat. It can be applied to herbs other than those included here but not St. John's wort as that needs light to work properly.
25g cayenne pepper
2 tablespoons of mustard powder
1 tablespoon of dried ginger
2 teaspoons of finely ground black pepper
300ml base oil of your choice
Blend the ingredients together and place in a heatproof container with a lid. Place this container into a pan of water which comes to 2cm below the rim. Heat the water and simmer for two hours. Allow the mixture to cool, strain through a fine cloth and store in a cool, dry place in an airtight container.

ointments

Ointments are made from oils or fats and incorporate waxes to thicken the mixture. Unlike creams they do not contain any water and are thick and greasy in texture. Their texture enables them to stay on the surface of the skin for a long time and is also especially good on very dry skin areas such as feet, knees and elbows.

They are generally quite warming preparations and are of great benefit for treating 'cold' conditions, such as rheumatism and deep aches. Their warming action makes them less suitable for 'hot' conditions such as psoriasis or inflamed or weeping skin conditions.

The wax element can be any wax, for example candle or paraffin wax, but my favourite is beeswax. Beeswax comes in two forms, bleached white or natural with its original honey colouring and smell. The oils can be plain, or infused oils such as Comfrey, Marigold, or St. John's wort. The oil element can be a base oil, a mix of different base oils, or an infused oil. Essential oils can be added to improve the scent, or as active medicinal ingredients.

simple ointment recipe
Using a ratio of 1 part wax to 10 parts oil, put the oil and wax into a heatproof bowl together. Place this bowl in a pan of water and slowly bring the water to the boil. When the water boils, turn the heat down to a gentle simmer and continue to heat and stir until the wax has dissolved completely then take off the heat. If you want to add essential oils, you do so at this point. Pour the ointment into the ointment containers, leave to set.

creams and lotions

Creams and lotions are emulsions of oil and water. Lotions are thinner than creams with a higher percentage of water. They both contain emulsifying agents to prevent the oil and water separating out but are more difficult to make than ointments as the oil and water parts sometimes separate with time. A bit of practice is needed to get the process perfected but once it is mastered there is an extensive range of ingredients to experiment with.

It is possible to use a commercially-produced base cream or lotion and add other herbal ingredients to it. The ingredients used to make up a base vary enormously and unfortunately many of the ingredients used, although totally legal, can be considered toxic. For example Butylparaben, a preservative used in many cosmetics, has recently been linked to oestrogenic cancers. There are other preservatives, collectively described as parabens (see glossary), which are not indicated in the same way. When making your own creams and lotions, as they are emulsions of fat and water and, as such, very easily infected if they are not prepared in a completely sterile environment, it is better to use a small amount of good quality parabens than to risk having an infected cream. I use products made by organic suppliers, like Aromantic (see Page 163), so I can be sure they will be the best quality and least damaging preservatives.

The amount of oil, tincture, tea or other product you want to add varies depending on the base you use. A bit of trial and error is required to get used to how the cream feels and reacts to added ingredients.

The first time you use a cream or lotion on someone and want to assess whether they are sensitive to it, use just 0.5% essential oil. That means 9 drops in a 60g jar. The essential oils are very strong and active at this seemingly low percentage. The highest percentage one should add is 5% but this would be for a very small area of the body, perhaps for use on a painful, arthritic joint.

I use infused oils and tinctures to a higher percentage, of up 10%. That means 6ml in a 60g jar of ointment. Alcohol can be drying to the skin so bear this in mind and avoid using tinctures if you are treating a dry skin problem.

The following recipes will help you get started on making creams and lotions but it is an enormous subject and if it seriously interests you there are courses dedicated to their production that are worth investigating. I would certainly recommend getting a good book, or researching information on the Internet to find out more.

making creams
You will need
Scales
2 measuring cylinders
2 mixing containers, heatproof
2 hot water baths, i.e. stainless steel saucepans
1 cold water bath, to allow the mixture to cool while being mixed
2 stainless steel or glass stirrers
1 handheld, electric mixer or whisk
1 spatula
1 or 2 thermometers (2 is best)
Two-ringed electric hotplate
Storage containers for the finished product

15g glyceryl sterate
10g cetyl alcohol
15g cocoa butter
22.5g sodium steroyl lactylate
45ml avocado oil
40ml thistle oil
315ml plain distilled water
15ml glycerine
10ml tocopherol
15ml natural deep moisturiser

Add glyceryl sterate, cetyl alcohol, cocoa butter, avocado oil and thistle oil to a mixing container. Set up your water bath on one of the rings of your hotplate and put the mixing container inside the water bath ready to heat.

Add sodium stearoyl lactylate, distilled water and glycerine into another container and heat alongside the first mixture over the second water bath. Both mixtures need to heat at the same rate so they reach approximately 75–80°C. Use the thermometers to check this.

Once they are at the correct temperature remove both mixtures from the heat. The next step is similar to mixing mayonnaise. Start to pour the oil mixture into the water mixture very slowly and patiently to avoid curdling and mix with the mixer. It should be held near the bottom of the container to avoid whisking in air, which will thicken the cream excessively.

Next, stand the container in the cold water bath to bring the temperature down to 40°C. Continue to whisk for five minutes. Set the mixer to a slow speed to keep the cream thinner or increase the speed to thicken it.

The spatula can also come in handy here to scrape the sides of the container intermittently. When the mix has reached 40°C more ingredients can be added: Natural deep moisturiser, preservative, such as parabens, if you are using one, vitamin E or CO_2 extracts. For this recipe we are adding only Natural deep moisturiser at this stage. At 25°C you can add essential oils or any other herbal components you do not want to be damaged by the heat. The mix can now be placed into the containers for storage. if you want to use a preservative such as parabens, use about 0.4–1%.

making lotions

The easiest way to make a lotion is to make a cream, as described above, and then add more sterilised water. To create a lotion from a cream add exactly the same volume of water as you have cream, so if you have 200ml cream add 200ml water. Use the mixer to blend as you slowly pour water into the mix.

Add essential oils to the cream before you blend more water in as they will mix much more smoothly at this stage. Other components can also be added to make the mix 'creamier' and less 'watery': add a further 3% glycerine and 2% Natural deep moisturiser as the water is blended in. More preservative may also be required so remember to increase the level to between 0.5–1% of the whole. When you have reached the right consistency put the lotion into the storage containers.

Using preservative in your product means it will keep, perhaps for as long as eighteen months. If you decide to include a preservative use about 0.4–1%. If you do not want to use one keep your creams and lotions in sterile containers, avoid any contamination, for example from dirty fingers, and keep it in a cool place such as a fridge.

essential oils

Essential oils can be blended or used singly and can be used in various ways.

baths add 5–10 drops to a bath, mix thoroughly or add a dispersing agent first, available from the suppliers listed (see Page 163).

inhalations useful for respiratory infections; use 2–3 drops in a bowl of hot, steaming water. Cover your head with a towel and inhale the steam. Be careful to close your eyes and do not breathe too deeply at first to avoid the hot steam irritating or burning the delicate membranes of the nose.

creams try at a low percentage, 0.5% (9 drops in 60g), to test for sensitivity to the oil then increase up to 3% as required. Increase this percentage to a maximum of 5% for small areas of treatment (90 drops in 60g). Stir the oil thoroughly into the cream.

massage oils test the oils at a low percentage for first usage as described for creams above and then use in the same proportions. The base oil could be an infused oil for added medicinal value; use St. Johns wort for nerve pain and spasm or Calendula and Comfrey for general healing. Stir the essential oils thoroughly into the base oil.

gels gel bases can be bought from suppliers, or you can grow your own Aloe vera plant and extract it yourself from the inner part of the leaf. The gel can be extracted simply by breaking off a leaf and squeezing the gel out. Gels are absorbed more quickly than oil or cream and are useful for applying essential oils to the skin in a diluted form when you require a speedy absorption, for example when treating arthritis of the hands and fingers a gel can be applied after washing and will be absorbed quickly so the hands are not left feeling greasy. Aloe gel has its own beneficial anti-inflammatory, cooling and healing properties which may also be utilised in this type of preparation. A gel for burns can be made using lavender essential oil added to aloe gel. The proportions of essential oils added should be the same as for creams. Oils do not mix easily with gels but will mix if you macerate them very well. Base oils, Infused oils, or essential oils and tinctures can be added.

essential oils Making your own is also possible, all you need is the herb to extract the oil from and a distillation kit. Distillation kits are commercially available for home use.

aromatic waters

Aromatic waters are wonderful taken internally as medicines or applied externally, and they can also be added to creams. If you are making creams from scratch they can be used as the water part of the cream mix.

It is also possible to make your own aromatic waters with the right equipment using a distillation kit. Distillation kits are commercially available for home use.

baths

Herbs can be added to the bath to relax both mind and body, treat infection and heal skin problems. Herbs can be used singly or a blend of herbs can be chosen to suit for medicinal reasons or for their scent.

My favourite bath blend is Lavender, Chamomile, Rose and Calendula. I use these herbs in combination for their general skin healing properties and also as they smell divine and encourage deep relaxation.
For each bath add 25g of herb to 2 litres of boiled water, infuse for 20 minutes, strain and add to the bath water.

cooking and eating herbs

There are many exciting ways to use herbs with food; here are just a few recipes to get you started.

lavender shortbread
Yields 12 shortbread
200g plain flour
2 tablespoons white rice flour or cornstarch
1 teaspoon dried lavender flowers (preferably English or French lavender)
⅛ teaspoon salt
100g unsalted butter, at room temperature
50g sugar and sugar for decoration
½ teaspoon lemon zest
½ teaspoon pure vanilla
Preheat the oven to 160°C.

Combine the flours, dried lavender and salt in a bowl; mix with a fork to blend. Mix the butter with the sugar until well blended then add the flavourings and the dry ingredients, mixing until just incorporated. Press into a 9-inch quiche pan (preferably with removable bottom) with the fingertips and score 12 wedges with the tines of a fork. Sprinkle with sugar. Bake in the lower third of the oven until the shortbread appears set when touched gently and is lightly coloured, which should be about 25 minutes. Cool on a rack for 10 minutes then cut into wedges. When almost cool remove from the pan with the aid of a small metal spatula.

note white rice flour is available in some supermarkets and health food shops.

angelica candy

Use Angelica stems and cut them into 4 inch lengths.

Steep the cut pieces in salt water for 12 hours.

Put a layer of cabbage or cauliflower leaves in a clean pan then a layer of Angelica, then a layer of leaves on top. Cover this with water and vinegar and boil it slowly until the Angelica becomes really green, then strain and retrieve the stems. Weigh the remaining stems.

Put an equal weight of sugar and place the sugar in a pan with enough water to allow it to dissolve. Bring the mixture to the boil then boil for ten minutes, stirring constantly, until it is fully dissolved. Pour the syrup over the Angelica stems and allow to stand for 12 hours. Then pour off the syrup, boil it again for 5 minutes and pour over the Angelica again. Repeat this process once more, then leave the Angelica in the sugar syrup and boil them both together until the Angelica becomes tender. Take the Angelica out of the sugar syrup, straining it through a sieve to remove the excess fluid. Sprinkle the stems with sugar to finish the candy and store in an airtight container for use as decoration on other sweets and desserts, or simply to eat as candy.

herb salad

1 handful of basil leaves, roughly torn
1 handful of coriander leaves, roughly torn
1 handful of sorrel, roughly torn

Chose several varieties of lettuce for their colour and texture, for example Lollo rosso, cos, romaine. Tear the lettuce and toss it with the herbs in a light sprinkling of olive oil and balsamic vinegar. Add salt and pepper to season.

nettle soup

2kg potatoes
1kg young nettles
30g butter
1litre chicken or vegetable stock
Sea salt and black pepper
100ml sour cream

Cook the peeled, chopped potatoes for 10 minutes in salted water. Drain. Wash and coarsely chop the nettles: only pick the new, young tops, and use gloves! Melt the butter in a saucepan, add the nettles and sweat them gently for a few minutes. Heat the stock and add to the nettles with the potatoes, bring to the boil and simmer for 10 minutes or until tender. Cool slightly and purée in a blender, adding seasoning and the sour cream. Reheat gently to serve.

herb gardening

what is a herb and a herb garden?

Herbs are defined as such by their use and significance to humans. They include plants valued as flavourings, dye, fibre, medicines and fragrances. Herbs are used in every area of life from the commercial to the spiritual world, where they are still commonly used in religious and spiritual ceremonies. A herb garden is, therefore, a garden created by growing a selection of plants which are useful. Whatever space or time you have for herb gardening there will always be a herb garden to suit you – whether it is a windowsill or an allotment, a patio or several acres of land.

herb growing through the ages

Some of the earliest herb gardens were planted about four thousand years ago in Egypt. Herbs used then are still recognised as having powerful medicinal actions today: Myrrh, Frankinsense, Fennel, Chamomile, Cassia and Senna.

The present, most popular, concept of a herb garden, an open space with divisions for different kinds of herbs, developed largely from ancient Egyptian, Islamic and Christian traditions. Within these traditions the garden was linked to a religious building or home, for example a monastery or temple, and the garden design would reflect the orderly style of the architecture and lifestyle and make economic use of space.

Early Christian Monasteries resembled Roman villas and inherited the Roman garden style which was geometric and formal. Plants found in a Roman garden would include Rosemary, Bay and Myrtle along with topiary and hedges.

Gardening became so important to the Benedictine order of monks that it came second only to prayer in their regime. A plan of a ninth century Benedictine monastery garden in Switzerland shows a rectangular garden with sixteen beds of herbs and a further, larger garden which contained vegetables and more herbs. Monasteries were largely self-sufficient and often relied on for medical assistance by the local communities and passing travellers. Their gardens reflected their responsibility for healing the sick. They also used herbs as flavourings and to produce ales, wines and liqueurs, for example Benedictine.

Herb gardening grew in popularity in Britain during the thirteenth century. Most large households had an extensive herb garden with a variety of herbs for both medicinal and culinary use.

In the sixteenth century, herbs were planted by universities that developed to teach botany and medicine: the two subjects were only separated in the eighteenth century. The demands of teaching influenced the layout of the gardens. In Edinburgh, for example, the herbs were planted in alphabetical order. As new species were brought back by explorers and traders the physic gardens, as they became known, expanded and have become the Botanic gardens we know today.

The seventeenth and eighteenth centuries saw a great change in style. Some of the finest formal herb gardens in the world were created in France, at châteaux such as Villandry, where they used box gardens to create their grand style. The potager style is also associated with this era. The first window boxes appeared in cramped Elizabethan London as a space-saving device.

Landscape gardening became fashionable during the eighteenth century and, as the industrial revolution progressed, the nostalgic, informal cottage garden style became popular.

Today there is an eclectic approach, choosing formal and informal as taste and space permits.

designing and creating a herb garden

A herb garden can be any size or shape; it does not necessarily have to be in a sunny, open position. There are herbs that will thrive in shade and in heavy wet ground, and some in water. The most popular type of herb garden is a small bed or border of culinary herbs within easy reach of the kitchen.

You could choose to have a herb garden devoted to medicinal herbs or exotics from around the world, to grow just one genus, or, perhaps, grow herbs which would be found in a monastic garden.

The main question to ask yourself is how much maintenance you are prepared to give to the plants. The answer determines how big the garden is, whether or not to garden in containers, whether to make it very formal or opt for a 'wild' look, and what kind of plants to use: annuals, perennials, tender perennials, or a mixture. Of course, budget plays a big part in this, too. The easiest to design, plant, and maintain is a small space, especially if you are new to gardening. A 2–3 metre square or round garden will suffice. You can always expand it or change the shape as it grows and your knowledge increases.

Another question to consider is where to put the garden. If you are growing a culinary herb garden I suggest you look out of your kitchen window for a suitable spot as close to the door as possible. If you want to pick herbs all year round ensure you create a suitable pathway, or use stepping stones to give good access in muddy weather. If container gardening is your thing, a sunny deck or patio is an ideal spot.

Start by sitting down with a pen and paper and make a few notes on the conditions at the chosen spot: soil type, wind, sun, shelter and any problems you have identified, such as a tree overhanging (not suitable for thymes but great for hops). This will enable you to choose the right herbs for your plot. Choose the herbs you want— you can always move plants around when you get them— but read the labels on the plants to judge how far apart to put them and how tall they will get to make sure low-growing plants get enough light.

You will find cultivation details for each herb featured in the Herb section of this book, starting on Page 61, but it is also worth checking with your supplier to get any other specific information on the herbs you purchase as there are many varieties available, all with possible slight variations in their preferences for position and soil type.

To create the shape required for your garden design you can use stakes and string or, if the design has a curvature, use a garden hose to make the outline. Then simply dig the garden, add some compost or well rotted-manure and you are on the way to a fantastic new herb garden. If there is any hard landscaping involved in your design, like brickwork or decking, then it is best laid prior to planting to avoid damage to the plants.

some designs to inspire

the formal herb garden
On a large scale this style of garden involves considerable quantities of hedging plants and paving thereby increasing the expense and amount of work required to get the project under way. However they are very easy to plant up and look interesting from the moment they are completed: unlike informal borders which rely on the plants for effect. It is a very practical way of managing the herb garden and dividing the herbs up into separate areas. Each section may have a theme, perhaps one section for heart herbs another for lung herbs ands so on, as seen in the Chelsea Physic Garden in London. Alternatively this structure can be used to separate out colours or you might alternate different coloured herbs within a bed to create dramatic, contrasting effects.

colour wheel with raised beds
Growing herbs in raised beds was a feature of Medieval and Renaissance times and the practice has been revived in recent times. It allows for better drainage, which is great for Mediterranean herbs such as Lavender and Rosemary. The other advantage of having raised beds is that the herbs are easier to access so they are simpler for anyone who has difficulty working at ground level to maintain, such as the elderly or anyone in a wheelchair. Gardeners with impaired vision may wish to add a scented or textured theme to the design with, perhaps, silky marshmallow and spiky houseleek among the sage and thyme.

In the following list there are three sizes of plant in each colour category so you can add or restrict height and depth as you wish and depending on the size of your garden.

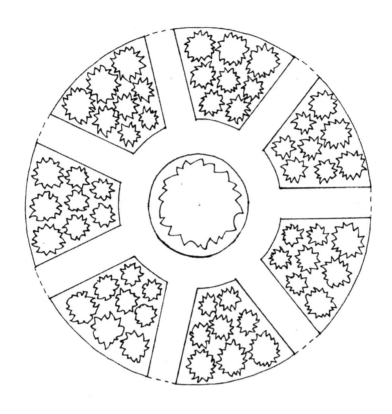

Central feature bay tree, orange or lemon tree,

purple
large Globe artichoke
medium Echinacea purpurea, Purple sage
small Skullcap, Verbena,

pink
large pink Hawthorn 'Paul's scarlet' (Crategus laevigata)
medium Rose (Rosa damscena)
small Soapwort, pink Yarrow

red
large Hibiscus
medium Bearberry (Arctostaphylos uva ursi)
small Corn Poppy (Papaver rhoeas)

orange
large Orange tree
medium Marigold, Californian poppy
small Pleurisy root

yellow
large Elecampane
medium St. John's wort, Evening primrose,
small Primula, Chamomile

green
large Gingko
medium Valerian, Fennel
small *Alchemilla mollis*, Thymus (white flowering)

blue
large Eucalyptus
medium Rosemary, Mallow 'Cottenham blue'
small Lavender, American liverwort (*Hepatica nobolis*),

informal wild herb garden

Many medicinal and culinary herbs originate from a wild habitat, and are also beautifully ornamental. They thrive in most garden conditions although some prefer more shade than others so check individual plants to see if they are suitable for the site you are working with. They love a well-drained, humus-rich soil.

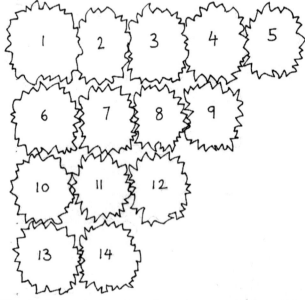

Plant scheme
1. Elderflower
2. Angelica archangelica
3. Gingko biloba
4. Lemon balm
5. Fennel
6. Echinacea purpurea
7. Verbena officinalis
8. Thyme
9. Motherwort
10. Mallow
11. Purple sage
12. Rosemary
13. Yarrow
14. Lavender

herbs in containers

Herbs work well in containers as the soil conditions each herb needs can be re-created, so the Mediterranean herbs get great drainage and the woodland herbs have their humus-rich soil. If your garden includes steps or a balcony, a collection of interesting containers can be layered for artistic effect. Hanging baskets can be used and climbers trained on special trellises designed for pots.

Window boxes are a great way to grow culinary herbs and, if you have room on your kitchen windowsill, they can be so convenient. The plants may get crowded in time and need replanting but they are worth saving and planting in larger containers or in the ground.

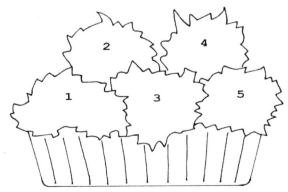

plant scheme
1. Thyme
2. Bay laurel
3. Rosemary
4. Purple sage
5. Lavender

To summarise: the first step is to think about where you would like the herb garden and make a note of the plot's features. For example how much sunlight it gets each day, whether it's north or south facing and so on. Measure the area and draw a basic plan. Then you can start to choose the type of herbs that will grow best in that space. Don't be afraid to make mistakes, experiment and find out what does and doesn't work for you and your garden. Try something new every year to keep your gardening exciting.

gathering, drying and storing herbs

gathering

Whether you are foraging for herbs out in the wild or collecting them from your own garden, gathering medicinal herbs is very satisfying. There are many written resources about when to collect medicinal herbs; some are based on up-to-date research on the chemistry of the plant and some are based on astrology or other, more ethereal ideas. To make sure you gather exactly what you intend to, particularly from the wild, it is a good idea to use a reliable field guide and I recommend *The Wild Flower Key: A Guide to Plant Identification in the Field, With and Without Flowers* by Francis Rose for this purpose (see Page 166 for full details).

As a general rule the level of active constituents is usually highest at the end of the period of most active growth. The medicinal plants should therefore be collected just before blossoming unless of course it is the ripe flowers or fruits you need.

Choose a dry day, one which has been sunny since daybreak is ideal, let the day progress enough so that the dew has lifted and there is as little moisture as possible in the atmosphere.

Dry the herbs in a warm, shady place. Not too hot as many herbs have medicinal essential oils in them which you want to retain. The temperature should be no higher than 35°C.

Pick only the best parts of the plant, the parts which are greenest and have not been affected by insect attack or other pathogenic factors. The stems or leaves should be cut with a sharp knife or scissors to prevent excess physical damage to the remainder of the plant and to encourage healthy growth to continue and prevent infection.

Many herbs grow in in abundance on wasteland and this can be taken advantage of. However, avoid using herbs which grow next to busy roads and may contain large amounts of pollutants, anything grown on any contaminated land or near the edges of fields which are sprayed with chemicals, pesticides, herbicides and fertilizers, as these will remain on the plant once dried and will be taken into the body easily when they are used as medicines.

Do investigate your local woodland and common land areas for herbs. If you have a local organic farm you may be able to investigate the hedgerows and pathways for medicinal herbs – with the farmer's permission of course.

drying herbs

Herbs are best dried by spreading them out in thin layers on a flat surface with good air circulation around them. Wire cooling racks from the kitchen are ideal for this purpose, or you can make your own with a bit of ingenuity. The amount of time required varies depending on the herb and the environment.

Check the herb regularly and rotate the plant matter to encourage thorough drying. Some herbs can be tied in bunches and hung from the ceiling to dry. To prevent dust collecting on them cover with a brown paper bag. If you choose to dry herbs like this make sure that the air is warm and has good circulation as it is less effective than the first method described but perhaps produces a more aesthetically pleasing product.

drying roots

Roots are more difficult to dry as they are generally collected during the damp days of autumn, when the soil is wet, sticky and muddy.

The ideal time to collect roots is after the leaves have died back and the nutrients have been sent to the roots for storage. This is the time when they are most potent. Use a spade or fork to lift the root so that the whole root is unearthed. If you want to grow the plant again the following season, divide the root, replant what you need and keep the rest to store and use.

The root you have collected needs to be cleaned thoroughly and scrubbing may be required to remove all residues. Any tops of the herb should be cut off and discarded (or composted). Some herbs are cut or split into 2 or more pieces to aid drying, for example,. Comfrey.

The roots should be spread out evenly on drying racks, or hung singly in a warm shed or greenhouse for about ten days. The root does not need to be dried in shade like aerial parts. The roots should shrivel over the first few days to about three-quarters of their original size, due to water loss. At this stage they can be dried in a cool oven or stacked above a stove so that warmer air can completely dry the root. If you use an oven set it to its coolest temperature, usually 110°C, and dry for a couple of hours, checking every half an hour or so as different roots dry at different rates. Once the roots are dry enough to store they should be quite brittle. Bulbs and corms can be dried like onions – tied into bunches in a shed, and checked regularly to ensure they are drying evenly.

storage

Once the plant material is completely dry it should be stored immediately. The ideal way to store herbs is in airtight containers made from glass, ceramic or metal. Plastic can be used but may absorb the essential oil aroma from scented herbs. They should also be stored away from sources of heat, moisture and direct sunlight.

Label the container with the name of the herb stored and the date it was collected. It is very easy to forget what herb was in which container, and dried, chopped herbs can look very similar. The date helps you to gauge how old the herb is and some dried herbs last longer than others. Myrrh lasts practically forever but most leaves and flowers are best used within a year of picking.

Similarly, essential oils should be stored away from heat, moisture and light as they are prone to oxidation and the products formed as a result can be irritating to the skin and mucous membranes.

glossary

adaptogen helps the body adapt to the stresses it is undergoing. It works to aid elimination and assimilation to make the body generally more effective.

alterative cleaning and nourishing herbs, they alter the condition of a tissue, detoxify polluted areas and help to restore the proper, healthy functioning of body tissues.

alkaloid these are organic substances which are usually obtained from plant matter. They have a bitter taste and some are toxic. They have a direct action on the body's tissues, mostly the nerves and blood vessels. Many herbs contain alkaloids including Comfrey and Passion flower. They are nitrogen-containing compounds that are physiologically active as drugs.

analgesic pain relieving.

anthelmintic eliminates parasitic worms from the intestines.

anticatarrhal helps to reduce catarrh production.

anticoagulant a substance that prevents blood clotting.

anticonvulsant a drug (or herb) used to prevent the severity of epileptic attacks.

antidepressant relieves symptoms of depression, usually mildly tonic in action.

antiemetic helps to reduce feelings of nausea and prevent vomiting.

anti-haemorrhagic stops blood flow.

antihistamine helps to reduce the inflammatory response associated with a histamine reaction, this includes the relief of itching sensations.

anti-inflammatory herbs which help to reduce inflammation. They often do not just act as symptomatic relief but also help the body to overcome the causes.

antilithic dissolves stones or gravel in the kidneys or gall bladder.

antimicrobials herbs which work directly on pathogens which may be the cause of disease, or they to increase the immune response so the body can fight the disease more effectively.

anti-neoplastic inhibits and combats the development of tumours

antirheumatic herbs which work to relieve the problems associated with rheumatism. An antirheumatic herb might have one or more action: it could aid elimination, reduce inflammation, increase circulation or relieve pain.

antiseptic works to clear any form of pathogenic infection.

antispasmodic reduces cramping and spasms in the muscle tissues of the body.

antitussive a respiratory relaxant used when the muscles involved in breathing become tense or strained through excessive coughing or overexertion.

anxiolytic mildly sedative like the nervine relaxants but they also have the specific action of relieving anxiety and any associated symptoms, for example palpitations.

aperitive encourages a healthy appetite

astringent helps to condense or tighten skin and mucosal tissue by causing a contraction in individual cell walls.

bitter stimulates the production of bile and often called cholagogues. Some are also called choleretics, which means they stimulate the release of bile from the gall bladder.

calminative calming to the nervous system.

carminative tones and relaxes the digestive system to help reduce production of wind and bloating by encouraging elimination of excess wind.

cephalic raises the blood circulation to the tissues of the head and brain.

cholagogue stimulates the production of bile by the liver.

choleretic stimulates the release of bile from the gall bladder, aiding digestion of fats.

circulatory stimulant aids the circulation in general and specifically the peripheral circulation.

co$_2$ extract an aromatic oil extracted using CO_2 – otherwise known as liquid carbon dioxide.

contraindications circumstances in which a particular herb should not be used, or should be used with caution.

demulcent provides a soothing effect on the mucous membranes

diaphoretic helps the body to sweat and break a fever.

digestive tonic stimulates the digestive functions of the body.

diuretic helps the body eliminate excess water and water soluble toxins via the kidneys.

diverticulas a pouch or sac branching out from a hollow organ or sac, usually pertaining to the intestine.

emmenagogue a herb which encourages delayed menstruation and help to regulate periods.

emollient softening substance applied to the skin.

epicarp the outermost layer of the pericarp (skin) of fruits.

evacuant promotes healthy bowel function and relieves constipation.

expectorant helps the lungs to expel more mucus.

galatogogue encourages milk flow in lactating women.

haemostatic helps stop the flow of blood where required for example in a nose bleed

hepatic a tonic for the liver function. They are also often bitters and cholagogues. Some hepatics can work to strengthen and protect the liver cells from toxins.

histamine hormones released as a response to allergens such as pollens. They negotiate the inflammatory response in bites and stings and the over-secretion of mucus in hayfever.

hypotensive reduces blood pressure.

immune stimulants are believed to increase the immune response to disease. Some herbs may act as immune system balancers so they can work effectively in helping treat auto-immune disorders.

indications circumstances in which a particular herb should be used.

laxatives encourage healthy bowel function and relieve constipation.

macerate extraction of the medicinal properties of the herb using a solvent, usually alcohol but also oil and water.

menorrhagia excessively heavy bleeding experienced during menstruation.

mucolytic breaks up thick mucus so it can be expelled more easily.

nervine herbs which have a positive effect on the nervous system.

nervine relaxant helps the mind and body to relax.

nervine stimulant stimulates the nervous system.

nervine tonic 'feeds' and strengthens a depleted nervous system, perhaps damaged by trauma, overwork and stress.

oedema an accumulation of bodily fluid, under the skin or within a body cavity.

orexigenic having a stimulating effect on the appetite.

parabens the collective term for a group of chemicals, including phenoxyethanol, methylparaben, ethyparaben, butylparaben and propylparaben, used as a preservative in the manufacture of herbal products like creams and lotions. Butylparaben has recently been linked to oestrogenic cancers so should be avoided.

parturient encouraging the onset of labour, child birth.

portal circulation the circulation that takes the blood from the stomach to the liver.

plasma the fluid in which blood cells are suspended.

prophylactic preventative medicine.

rubefacient these products are applied to the skin, rather than taken internally. They heat the area, increasing circulation, relieving congestion and reducing inflammation. They are very powerful in effect and should not be used internally or on broken or damaged skin.

sialogogue increase saliva production.

steroidal has an action on the body of a steroid.

stomachic a tonic for the stomach's function.

styptic contracting the tissues or blood vessels, astringent. Sometimes this also refers to stopping bleeding by contracting the tissues or blood vessels.

uterine tonic strengthens and tones the tissues and function of the reproductive organs, in both in males and females.

vasodilator widens the blood vessels as a result of relaxing the muscles of the blood vessels walls.

volatile alkaloid a volatile compound, like an essential oil, which evaporates easily.

vulnerary a plant which has a cleansing and healing effect on a wound. They are thought to increase the rate of cellular regeneration which, in turn, increases the speed of healing, and encourages the immune system response in the local area.

herbal remedies: how to make, use and grow them **L I L I**

resources

herb, medicine and product suppliers

The Medicine Garden
Low Impact Living Initiative (LILI) online shop
Redfield
Winslow, Bucks
MK18 3LZ
www.lowimpact.org
+44(0)1296 714184

The Organic Herb Trading Company
Milverton
Somerset, TA4 1NF
www.organicherbtrading.com
info@organicherbtrading.com
+44(0)1823 401205, fax +44(0)1823 401001

Avicenna
Bidarren
Cilcennin
Lampeter
Ceredigion
Wales SA48 8RL
avicenna@clara.co.uk
+44(0)1570 471 000

G. Baldwin & Co
171/173 Walworth Road
London SE17 1RW
sales@baldwins.co.uk
+44(0)207 703 5550, fax +44(0)207 252 6264

Aromantic Ltd
17, Tytler Street
Forres
Moray IV36 1EL
www.aromantic.co.uk
+44 (0)1309 696900, fax +44 (0)1309 696911

herbalists

Sorrell Robbins BSc(Hons), MNIMH, MCHyp, MABCH, MIFPA
The Medicine Garden,
93 Ringstead Road,
London SE6 2BT
07814 430690
sorrellrobbins@gmail.com

National Institute of Medical Herbalists
56 Longbrook Street
Exeter
Devon EX4 6AH
www.NIMH.Org.UK
+44(0)1392 426022

jars & bottles

Wains of Tunbridge Wells Ltd
Tunbridge Wells Enterprise Centre
Chapman Way
North Farm Road
Tunbridge Wells
Kent TN2 3DU
+44(0)1892 521666, fax +44(0)1892 515334

Bottle Company (South) Ltd.
Broadmead Lane
Keynsham
Bristol BS31 1ST
+44(0)117 986 9667, fax 0117 986 6335
www.bottlecompanysouth.co.uk

capsule and pessary making equipment

Quaestus
1 Castle Meadows
Abergaveny
Wales NP7 7RZ
+44(0)1873 85299. fax +44(0)1873 859399

essential oils

Essentially Oils Ltd
8 Mount Farm
Junction Road
Churchill
Chipping Norton
Oxon OX7 6NP
www.essentiallyoils.com
+44(0)1608 659544, fax +44(0)1608659566

Materia Aromatica
7 Penrhyn Crescent
London SW14 7PF
www.materia-aromatica.com
sales@materia-aromatica.com
Tel: +44 (0) 20 8932 9868

courses

Residential weekend course: herbal medicine, at LILI, www.lowimpact.org. +44(0)1296 714184.

information

The Herb Society
PO Box 626
Banbury
Oxon OX17 1XB
www.herbsociety.co.uk
Tel: + 44 1295 812 376
LILI forum at http://www.lowimpact.org/forums/

books

These books are all available from LILI

The Wild Flower Key: A Guide to Plant Identification in the Field, With and Without Flowers
Francis Rose
Frederick Warne Publishers Ltd
An excellent guide for identifying herbs: highly recommended.

Herbal Remedies
Christopher Hedley & Non Shaw
Parragon
A practical, beginner's guide to making effective remedies in the kitchen.

The New Holistic Herbal
David Hoffman
HarperCollins Publishers Ltd
A practical guide to using herbal remedies for healing.

Encyclopedia of Herbal Medicine
Thomas Bartram
Grace Publishers
A comprehensive A–Z of diseases and corresponding herbal treatments.

A Modern Herbal
Mrs M. Grieve
Penguin Books Ltd
The medicinal, culinary, cosmetic and economic properties, cultivation and folklore of herbs, grasses, fungi, shrubs and trees.

The Complete Women's Herbal
Anne McIntyre
Gaia Books Ltd
A manual of healing herbs and nutrition for personal wellbeing and family care.

British Herbal Pharmacopoeia
British Herbal Medicine Association
233 Monographs of herbs with details of medicine making.

The Herb Society's Complete Medicinal Herbal
Penelope Ody
Dorling Kindersley Publishers Ltd
A beautifully presented, practical guide to medicinal herbs with remedies for common ailments.

The Complete Herbal
Nicholas Gent Culpeper
Wordsworth Reference

The Complete Herbal
Nicholas Gent Culpeper
http://www.bibliomania.com/2/1/66/113/frameset.html
The complete text online.

notes